The Healthy Truth

Biblical Principles for Wellness

Lesa Lawson, ND

The Healthy Truth
Biblical Principles for Wellness

ISBN-13: 978-1979319249
ISBN: 1979319243

For Thaddeus – your ailment has been a
revelation to us both, and with careful thought, I
helped you pack for your journey.
Here is your remedy chest. Signs, wonder,
lessons, and musings are contained therein. The
prospect of seeing you fully recovered fills me with
a curious pleasure, so there is also
the joy of discovery.
Explore, experiment, and recover your health.
There is yet room in the chest for your pledge.

LET IT BE UNDERSTOOD

The standard disclaimer is simply this: the information contained in this book is not intended to provide medical advice nor should it take the place of medical treatment from your own physician.

That disclaimer, however, is antithetical to my purpose. I have written to encourage people to think critically and do for themselves what no physician can do.

The author does not take responsibility for any consequence from any remedy or application of supplements, herbs or preparations by any person reading the information in this book.

CONTENTS

I ACKNOWLEDGE

Without apology, my Lord and Savior Jesus Christ, the One whose healing of my body strengthened me to rediscover a better way of living and regain my health. In regaining my health, I am empowered to help others in the recovery of their own.

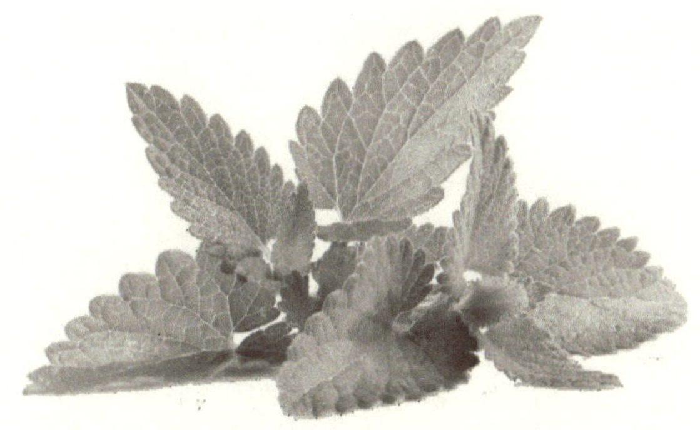

You have held me accountable, family, friends, clients; even conversationalists in lines at the supermarket. Now, I return the favor, bestowing culpability upon you through this book. Please feel free to accept every measure of responsibility.

Body Signals (A Witty Ditty)

Lesa Lawson

My body's on loan to me and experience has shown
that the payments and upkeep, they are mine alone
I've learned a hard lesson, so, I now take great care
to maintain it; yes, keep it from trauma and wear
The first years that I had it were really a breeze
I relied on my dad and my mom with great ease
They nurtured, I enjoyed; they fed me - what bliss!
Then I grew older; I became a "big miss".

Hmm, that was ok, though, I decided then,
since they still took care of me:
dad - provider, mother - hen
Then I became a teenager and thought I was grown
so, they kept pulling back 'til I was doing it alone
Now, I'm free, I kept thinking, I can take care of me
What a crock! I found that out. I'll tell you – you'll see

Well, I ate what I wanted and more and more, too
I ate junk – no one could tell me what I could not do
Adult, now, and working, I could try anything:
pizza, ice-cream, Chinese - pick it up, order in.

I explored all food kinds and flushed them with drink
of all flavors and colors – milky, carbonated, blue, green,
pink

I even mixed drinks with alcohol, and one specialty
was to mix drinks and name them like some royalty

Well, one day, I noticed a twinge in my gut
or thought I did anyway, and shrugged it off, but
it persisted, with headaches; not too badly at first,
then, growing in intensity, with nausea – the worst
Constant pain, colds aplenty, a bad combination
Skin grew blotchy; lips grew dark,
then moodiness, depression.

Didn't make the connection, didn't notice the trend
Then something happened, the beginning? The end?

I bought a rump roast and called up my mom
to ask how to cure it and roast it; yum yum!
She gave careful instructions, I took careful note
to follow them, I couldn't wait for the slide down my throat
It smelled oh, so heavenly, I sat with my plate
and my knife at the ready; oh, I had a date!

At long last, 'twas ready; I cut a thick slice
Juices flowed forth, browned perfection
I didn't even want rice
Beef slid into my mouth, tender, juices like wine
I prepared to enjoy more. Oh joy! 'twas all mine!

Ten minutes of joy later, I felt the first heave
and ran to the toilet, there my roast beef to leave

I left it and left it and when I was through
I'd befriended the toilet; beef no longer drew

Roast beef reeked in my apartment, the smell made me hurl
My head strongly protested, my insides awhirl
Into the garbage went the pan and pot roast
but the smell of it lingered like a proverbial ghost
For days, I would dry-heave because of the smell
and it finally came home to me that all was not well

Well, so much has happened since then, but I've learned
that while I experimented, my body discerned
that I needed to return to the way I was raised;
eating foods that would benefit, instead of being crazed
Processed foods, they don't benefit, they are just designed
to put your body in nutritional debt, just like mine

If you're getting signals from your body at all
don't ignore them; you're setting yourself up for a fall
Your body will tell you when all is not well
Take heed and learn from my small taste of hell

INTRODUCTION

When the body's not well
It affects all we do
Sickness is a great yoke
Those afflicted will tell you

How can people who are alive and supposedly well, be rotting? We have more gyms, more food and a great variety of it too, in our western part of the world. We have some of the best doctors, hospitals, and medical equipment. Why then, are we so sick? Why are we weakened, despite the many medications and supplements that we take? Why do we smell like rotting meat, when we eat some of the best meals that money can buy?

Dirty – Inside and Out

Illness is a household name in our nation, appearing in so many forms, and craftily concealing itself beneath the covers of accepted terminology, like migraines, reflux disease, celiac disease, nasal and respiratory allergies, stomach pain, and cancer, to name a few.

The stage is set: baby to toddler, hopefully eating wholesome, fresh foods that caregivers can provide. Yet, even at this early stage, there lurks a devil: margarine or cheese on the vegetables, pasteurized whole milk from hormone-blitzed cows, and sugar-sweetened drinks. These substances (for I cannot call them food) begin to deplete and denature our supply of enzymes, rendering them unable to perform. One function of enzymes is to help to digest food.

By the time we reach adulthood, the enzyme supply is depleted, if the food choices remain poor. The body struggles to digest food, some of which it has begun to regard as foreign matter. Heartburn and other digestive ailments begin to surface, which lead to other ailments. With the influx of more chemicals into our food, our children are also being assaulted by some of these symptoms, among them reflux issues, stomach pain, constipation, and diabetes.

We have become lost on the road of good health. Where did we veer? We must return to the beginning to find answers to many of the illnesses from which we suffer. I, by no means, am saying that we will live forever or that illness may never strike. Indeed, we have done so much harm to ourselves that we should be immensely thankful to the One who made our bodies in such a way, that they can fall back on defensive measures, at least for a time. Defensive measures, should, after all, be temporary. If left to exist in defense mode, the body will eventually stop working.

In an age where we are inundated with so much information and choices, many of us do nothing because we do not know what to do. Unbeknownst to many, the

Bible offers clear instructions on how we ought to live, not only spiritually but also physically, emotionally, and even financially. Careful perusal of its pages and, more importantly, adherence to its guidelines will prove beneficial and life-changing. A guidebook on the body given to us directly from the Maker of the body – what better guide is there?

CHAPTER 1

IN THE BEGINNING – DIETARY 101

The introduction to the undisputed, phenomenal masterpiece – and I am not talking about this book. The Bible's first book of Genesis details the creative genius of God, Master Architect, Builder, Counselor, and Nutritionist. Chapter 1:11-12 document that God created, on the third day, *"seed-bearing plants and trees on the land… according to their various kinds… and God saw that it was good."* Note: the plants all had seeds.

On the sixth day, after God had created man, his highest, and most intelligent creation, God said to Adam,

"And God said, "Behold, I have given you every plant yielding seed that is on the face of all the

earth, and every tree with seed in its fruit. You shall have them for food." Genesis 1:29

There is a wide variety of fruits, vegetables, grains, spices, and herbs that are detailed in the Bible, each providing vital nutrients that amply sustained the people who lived, then, and continue to do so, now. Each food kind is mentioned deliberately because of the host of vitamins, minerals and phytochemicals contained therein.

Phytochemicals, according to cancer.org, are the extensive variety of compounds that are produced by plants. Fruits, vegetables, legumes, grains, and other plants are all sources of phytochemicals. Some of the more well-known phytochemicals are beta carotene, ascorbic acid (vitamin C), folic acid, and vitamin E. http://cancer.org/docroot/ETO/content/ET...

Many of these life-sustaining foods are listed in the following table:

Foods (non-meats) in the Bible

Almonds—Genesis 43:11; Numbers 17:8

Anise—Matthew 23:23

Apples—Song of Solomon 2:5; Joel 1:12

Barley—Ruth 2:23

Barley Bread—2 Kings 4:42

Beans or Pulse (Legumes)—2 Samuel 17:28

Bitter Herbs (dandelion greens, watercress, arugula, parsley, cilantro)—Exodus 12:8

Bread—Luke 22:19

Carob (St. John's Bread)—Matthew3:4; Mark 1:6

Cinnamon—Exodus 30:23

Coriander—Exodus 16:31; Numbers 11:7

Corn—Ruth 2:14; I Samuel 17:17

Cinnamon—Exodus 30:23; Revelations 18:13

Cucumbers—Numbers 11:5

Cumin or Cummin—Isaiah 28:25

Curds (Cottage and Ricotta Cheese)—Genesis 18:8

Dates—2 Samuel 6:19

Dill—Matthew 23:23

Dried Fruits—Genesis 3:2

Figs—Numbers 13:23; I Samuel 25:18

Flax Seed—Exodus 9:31

Flour (Whole Meal)—Ezekiel 16:19; Numbers 6:15

Fruits (All)—Genesis 1:29

Garlic—Numbers 11:5

Grapes—Deuteronomy 24:21

Grape Juice (New Wine)—Zechariah 9:17

Herbs (Leafy Plants) and Vegetables—Genesis 1:29; Proverbs 15:17

Herbs (Seasonings)—Proverbs 27:25; Matthew 13:32

Honey—Proverbs 24:13; Proverbs 25:16

Hyssop (Caper)—Psalms 51:7; John 19:29

Lamb and Sheep—Deuteronomy 14:4

Leeks—Numbers 11:5

Lentils—Genesis 25:34

Leaven (Yeast)—Leviticus 23:17; Galatians 5:9

Marjoram (Hyssop)—Exodus 12:22

Melon—Numbers 11:5

Millet—Ezekiel 4:9

Mint—Matthew 23:23; Luke 11:42

Mulberry—2 Samuel 5:24; 1 Corinthians 14:14

Mustard Seeds—Mark 4:31; Luke 13:19

Nuts—Song of Solomon 6:11

Olives and Olive Oil—Leviticus 2:4; Deuteronomy 8:8

Onions—Numbers 11:5

Pistachio Nuts—Genesis 43:11

Pomegranates—Numbers 13:23

Raisins—2 Samuel 16:1

Rye—Isaiah 28:25

Saffron—Song of Solomon 4:14

Salt—Leviticus 2:13; Luke 14:34

Sourdough Bread—Leviticus 23:17; Amos 4:5

Spelt (Fitches)—Ezekiel 4:9

Spices—1 Kings 10:10

Squash (Gourds)—2 Kings 4:39

Sweet Cane—Isaiah 43:24; Jeremiah 6:20

Unleavened Bread (Tortillas, Flat Bread, Chapattis)—Gen. 19:3; Exod. 29:2

Vinegar—Ruth 2:14

Water—Genesis 21:19; John 4:7

Wheat—Deuteronomy 32:13, Ruth 2:23; Psalm 81:16

Wheat bread—Exodus 29:2

Wine—John 2:1-10, 1 Timothy 5:23

Source: http://www.hillbillyhousewife.com/biblicalfoods.htm. 2012

Thus, began man's diet and he continued in this mode until after his sin of disobedience and subsequent fall.

Being ejected from the garden changed man's lifestyle and he began to work for his food, where before it was readily available. With the arduous labor and the *"sweat of the brow"* came additions to man's diet, after a time, in the form of meat. When God brought Noah and his family out of the ark, after he had cleansed the earth with the flood, he told them that *"…every moving thing that lives shall be meat for you; even as the green herb, have I given you all things."* Gen. 9:3-4

Animal flesh and fish were added to the diet at this point. God warned the Noahs, however, that animal flesh with the blood was not to be eaten because the blood is the life (the soul) of the creature. The blood had to be drained and covered or broiled out of the meat before it could be consumed.

Interestingly enough, up until this point, no mention

was made of illness; people seemed to die of old age, the result of the curse that Adam initiated.

Clean Meats of the Bible

Land Creatures
Cattle - Beef, Hamburger, Veal.
Sheep - Lamb, Mutton.
Others - Antelope, Buffalo (Bison), Caribou, Deer (Venison), Elk, Gazelle, Giraffe, Goat, Hart, Ibex, Moose, Reindeer, Locust.
Water Creatures
Anchovy, Bass, Bluefish, Carp, Cod, Flounder, Grouper, Grunt, Haddock, Halibut, Herring, Mackerel, Minnow, Perch, Pickerel, Pike, Rockfish, Salmon, Shad, Smelt, Snapper, Sole, Steelhead, Sunfish, Tarpon, Tuna (Albacore, Bonita, Yellowtail).
Air Creatures
Chickens, Dove, Duck, Goose, Grouse, Guinea Hen, Partridge, Peacock, Pheasant, Pigeon, Songbird, Sparrow, Quail, Turkey.

God's instruction to Noah and his family was the first time that meat was officially recorded as being eaten by man [Genesis 18].

Abram received three men in the plains of Mamre, as he sat in the tent door in the heat of the day. He sensed that these were not ordinary visitors. After beseeching and gaining their consent to dine with him, Abram instructed Sarah to make cakes out of fine meal. He then ran to the herd and selected *"a calf tender and good"* and gave it to a servant to be prepared into "savory meat" for their guests.

Abram's herd was not given growth hormones or injected with steroids and antibiotics; rather, this cattle owner adhered to God's instructions that were given to Adam so long ago, that *"to every beast of the earth, and to every fowl of the air, and to every thing that creeps upon the earth, wherein there is life, I have given every green herb for meat." Genesis 1:30.*

Abram's cattle, as with all herds of the Jewish people, was able to graze on hillsides and plains. They meandered among lush, verdant greenery, watched over by shepherds. Those cattle were what would now be considered "range-free."

CHAPTER 2

SPLITTING HAIRS AND HOOVES

As the children of Israel grew in number and began to develop a personality among other nations, God provided detailed instructions regarding their diet. They would need to learn to maintain their way of eating when among these other nations. These instructions, if we were to follow them today, would prove quite beneficial. In Leviticus 3:17, for example, God reminded them that they should not eat meat with blood in it, neither should they eat a certain kind of fat.

The forbidden fat is that which surrounds the vital organs and the liver. The Jewish Virtual Library states that present day scientists have discovered that there are biochemical differences between the forbidden fat and the permissible fat around the muscles and under the skin. If we were to consider this, we would realize that certain types of fat are the cause of many of our heart disease and diabetes issues.

There is fat that is permissible to eat; this fat is translated as the "oil of the olive," according to Dr. Rex Russell. (*Healthy Living*, p.68). In addition, the fat of nuts, seed, fruits, vegetables, and legumes are most healthful and therefore allowed. Butter of kine (cows) and milk of sheep are also permitted.

Blood contains the life or soul of the animals; it should be drained, and the meat soaked, or the blood should be broiled away, completely removed from the meat. Fish, though not broiled, is also drained and cleaned of blood. Since removing the blood from fish is important to health, sushi, of the raw fish variety, presents a problem. Eating red meat in "rare" form is also an issue.

Consider also that the blood can contain parasites,

which transfer into the human body when consumed. Parasites wreak havoc on the body and can cause many illnesses, some of which can lead to death. Pigs are noted harbingers of parasites because of their lack of discrimination regarding that which they eat.

The Food and Agriculture Organization of the United Nations noted that pigs can be infected with Trichinella from eating rats which have that infection. According to Dr. Rex Russell, a study of Egyptians revealed that they contained "eggs from Schistosoma, Trichinella, wire worm and tape worms, all of which are found in pork. All of these organisms cause significant chronic diseases." Pigs eat garbage and sometimes, even their own young, dead or alive. Mange and worms from pigs can cause disease in humans. Rabbits, another 'no-no' animal for food can cause tularemia (an infectious disease) in humans.

The eleventh chapter of Leviticus provides the most detailed information on dietary regulations. God said that the children of Israel could eat flesh but not all kinds. They could eat *"whatsoever parts the hoof, and is cloven-footed, and chews the cud"*; but of the beasts that chew the cud, they were not allowed to eat those that did not fulfill all requirements, like the camel, coney (rock badger), hare and swine. (verses 4-7)

Any product that is derived from these unclean animals is forbidden. Gelatin, therefore, which is usually made from the hooves of horses, is on the list. Unfortunately, it is used in many foods, some of which we may know, but others may be a surprise. Gelatin is used in dairy products such as sour cream, yogurt, and buttermilk; in desserts like Jell-O, marshmallows, icing, glazes and cream fillings, mousse, and whipped toppings; in jellied meats, such as consommé; in wines, canned ham, and in nutritional and pharmaceutical products.

Gelatin is also used in non-edible products like carbonless copy paper, cosmetics such as lipsticks and nail polish, and in hair products. If we are unaware that gelatin is in these things that we consume, we need to start paying closer attention, as we are bringing sickness upon our unsuspecting bodies.

Rennet is an enzyme that is used to harden most cheeses, and is often obtained from the stomach lining of the animals forbidden for meat. It would, then, be unclean, making most cheeses unclean. That is certainly something to consider regarding our abundant consumption of most hard and "non-kosher" cheeses.

Some insects were allowed for meat in the Bible but as the years progressed, confusion ensued, in the Jewish faith, as to which were considered clean, therefore they have all been forbidden. For most of us, this is not an unpleasant notion; still, we may not realize that many food additives and food colorings are made from insects. The FDA, in its Code of Federal Regulations Title 21, stated that carmine, the red dye used in foods and make-up, is made from cochineal bugs.

In addition to those forbidden creatures, all crustaceans and any other sea creature that does not have scales and fins are unclean and forbidden; in fact, God called them "an abomination." (Leviticus 11:9-12) Interestingly enough, these creatures are referred to as bottom feeders or scavengers. They eat refuse and other things equally unappealing. Our consumption of these creatures makes us vulnerable to the bacteria and diseases that they ingest. Scavengers of the air, like vultures, and birds of prey, like owls and hawks, are also included in this list.

List of Forbidden Foods in the Bible

<table>
<tr><td colspan="1">Land Creatures</td></tr>
<tr><td>

- **Swine** - Boar, Peccary, Pig (Hog), Bacon, Ham, Lard, Pork.
- **Canine** - Coyote, Dog, Fox, Hyena, Jackal, Wolf.
- **Feline** - Cat, Cheetah, Leopard, Lion, Panther, Tiger.
- **Equine** - Donkey, Horse, Mule, Onager, Quagga, Zebra.
- **Miscine Munimus** - Badger, Coney, Hare, Monkey, Opossum, Porcupine, Raccoon, Skunk, Squirrel.
- **Miscine Maximus** - Bear, Camel, Elephant, Gorilla, Hippo, Kangaroo, Lama, Rhino, Wallaby, Chevrotain.

</td></tr>
<tr><td>Water Creatures</td></tr>
<tr><td>

- **Fish** - Catfish, Eel, Marlin, Shark, Sturgeon.
- **Hard Body** - Abalone, Clam, Crab, Crayfish, Lobster, Mussel, Prawn, Oyster, Scallop, Shrimp.
- **Soft Body** - Cuttlefish, Jellyfish, Limpet, Octopus, Squid.
- **Sea Mammals** - Dolphin, Otter, Seal, Walrus, Whale.
- **Others** - Crocodile, Turtle, Frog, Newt, Salamander, Toad, Lizard.

</td></tr>
<tr><td>Air Creatures</td></tr>
<tr><td>

Albatross, Bat, Bittern, Condor, Cormorant, Crane, Crow, Cuckoo, Eagle, Flamingo, Grosbeak, Gull, Hawk, Heron, Kite, Lapwing, Loon, Osprey, Ostrich, Owl, Woodpecker, Pelican, Penguin, Plover, Raven, Stork, Swallow, Swan, Swift, Vulture, Water Hen.

</td></tr>
</table>

Adapted from Richard Anthony's Biblical Health Principles:
http://ecclesia.org/truth/health.html

CHAPTER 3

FOOD COMBINING

"Do not seethe (boil) a kid in its mother's milk." Exodus 23:19, 34:26, Deuteronomy 14:21

God issued this thrice-repeated directive to the children of Israel. He did not need to give an explanation, yet, over time, we have come to understand that the eating of meat with dairy in the same meal or timeframe interferes with digestion. The children of Israel already knew this because God told them. The modern world has learnt this lesson the hard way because we regard the dietary instructions in the Bible as being outdated.

The Jewish Virtual Library, as well as Jewfaq.org state that most Jews who observe the *kashrut* (biblical dietary restrictions) will wait for three to six hours after a meat meal before eating dairy products. This is done for digestive and separation purposes and also because there are remnants of meat or fat that tend to remain in the crevices of the mouth for several hours.

We now know that the body uses different enzymes to digest different foods. We also know that digestion issues occur when enzymatic activity is compromised or depleted. Unfortunately, many of us still have butter or rich, creamy sauces with meats, or hamburgers with milkshakes and the like. Continued eating of this kind may result in stomach pain and/or distention, as undigested foods rot (putrefy) within the digestive tract. Inflammation then occurs, leading to bigger problems. Heartburn can also result, as well as insulin resistance.

GENERAL RULES OF FOOD COMBINATION TO AID DIGESTION

Foods digest at different rates in the body, using different enzymes that are made in the body. Some foods are better assimilated in an acidic environment and others are broken down in a more alkaline environment. Several factors can interfere with the digestive process.

Drinking water with your meals dilutes the digestive fluids and inhibits assimilation.

Building vegetable salads with all sorts of fruits, nuts, seeds and dressings can also dilute and slow nutritional benefits. Meat with milk, processed foods with sugary drinks, and dairy with fruit add to digestive grief. Certain foods, when eaten in combination with other foods, do not digest well. Due to various transit times of food and the different digestive enzymes needed, you may be left feeling heavy, fatigued, bloated, and gaseous.

Because our bodies use different digestive

enzymes to digest different foods, when we eat certain foods together, the body must secrete or produce several different enzymes, simultaneously. Depending on the food combinations, this may place strain on the body.

In secreting these enzymes, the body creates different pH environments to facilitate digestion. If it is producing several enzymes, together, there is the possibility that digestion slows. Putrefying food starts depositing toxins into the body. The stored toxins and undigested, fermenting foods bring other problems, among them malabsorption, bad breath and other strong odors, low energy, poor sleep, and general ill-health.

There are simple rules concerning the combination of foods. The speed at which foods digest is something that must be considered. Fruits, for examples digest faster than all other foods. Proteins digest the most slowly. As such, we should consider this when preparing and eating meals. This allows our bodies to gain and use the nutrients in food.

In terms of digestion rates, then, it should be thus:

1. fruits
2. greens
3. non-starchy vegetables
4. starches
5. protein

Eating foods in the correct order (according to their transit times) ensures a traffic jam-free and healthy digestive tract.

Rules to Reconcile:

- **Maintain your digestive fluids.** Drinking water while eating neutralizes digestive fluids. Combining certain foods neutralizes stomach acidity, making it hard to break down acidic food. For examples, when protein and carbs are eaten together, digestion slows, thereby increasing the chances of indigestion.

Food combination rules:

- **Don't eat protein with carbohydrates.** Proteins digest well with vegetables, and carbohydrates digest well with vegetables.

- **Eat fruits only when they are ripe and when you are well.** If you are ill, limit fruit. Once you have regained optimum health, fruits can be reintroduced into your diet. Fruits contain sugar, and while sugar from fruits is more healthy than other sugars, sugar still feeds disease. Sugar causes stress to our pancreas, and when pancreatic function is lessened, our insulin levels fall, as well. Insulin is the hormone that transports sugar from the bloodstream to the body's cells.

- **Don't eat fruit and veggies together.** Fruits digest quickly and should be eaten on their own. Green leafy vegetables such as spinach, chard, collards are the only vegetables that digest well with fruits.

- **Eat melon by itself.** Melon has the highest sugar content of all fruits and should be eaten sparingly. Melons typically digest in about 20 minutes of eating. Because of its fast digestion time, if eaten with other foods melon will ferment, causing gas.

- **Don't restrict fast-digesting foods.** Eat first the foods that will digest the fastest. Mixing those with slow-digesting foods will impair the digestive process, causing bloating, gas, and poor nutrient assimilation.

If you are not sure where to start, pay attention to how you feel after a meal, especially one in which many types of foods are combined. After noting your food reactions for a few days, try different food combinations, based upon the list, and note whether you feel the difference.

Let's review for better digestion

1. Don't mix fruit with veggies, grains, or proteins. If combining fruits, don't mix acidic fruits with sweet fruits.

2. Don't mix carbohydrates and starches with proteins. Instead, combine carbohydrates and starchy foods with vegetables, and combine proteins with veggies.

3. Keep your meals simple. When combining veggies, try not to combine more than a few. All greens mix well with one another.

4. Avoid drinking with your meals. It dilutes the enzymes and your digestive fire.

5. Eat fast-digesting foods and raw foods, first before any cooked food or food that will take longer to digest.

FRUITS: **Should be eaten alone and on an empty stomach. They can be combined with raw leafy greens. Don't mix acidic with sweet.**

Melons Watermelon, Honeydew, Cantaloupe

Citrus Oranges, Grapefruit, Clementine

Exotic Fruit Papaya, Pineapple, Starfruit

Seeded Fruit Apples, Pears, Berries, Bananas

Pitted Fruit Cherries, Plums, Peaches, Avocados

DRIED FRUIT, NUTS and SEEDS: **Combine with bananas and raw vegetables. (Don't drink while eating.)**

Unsulphured Dried Fruit, Dried Apricots, Dried Apples

Raw Seeds and Seed Butters Sesame Seeds, Sesame Tahini, Sunflower Seeds, Chia Seeds

Raw Nuts and Nut Butters Almonds, Almond Butter, Cashews, Cashew Butter, Pecans, Brazil nuts

Seed Milks: Sesame Milk, Hempseed Milk

Nut Milks: Almond Milk, Hazelnut Milk

COOKED STARCHES: Combine with all raw and cooked vegetables and avocados.

Winter Squash Acorn, Butternut, Kabocha

Millet, Quinoa, Buckwheat, Kamut, Amaranth, Whole Grains, Rice,

Oats, Wheat berries, Bulgur, Sprouted Grain Baked Products,

Ezekiel Bread, Whole Grains, Whole Grain Cereals

ANIMAL FLESH/ PROTEIN: Combine with all raw vegetables and cooked non-starchy vegetables.

Raw Goat, Cow and Sheep Cheese, Pecorino Pasteurized Goat and

Sheep Cheese, Chevre, Feta, Mozzarella

Wild-caught Fish: Halibut, Cod, Salmon, Sole

Game: Venison, Bison, Grass-Fed Beef

LEGUMES: Combine with all raw and cooked vegetables, cooked starches and grains, and avocados.

Beans: Kidney, Pinto, Garbanzo, Navy, Lima

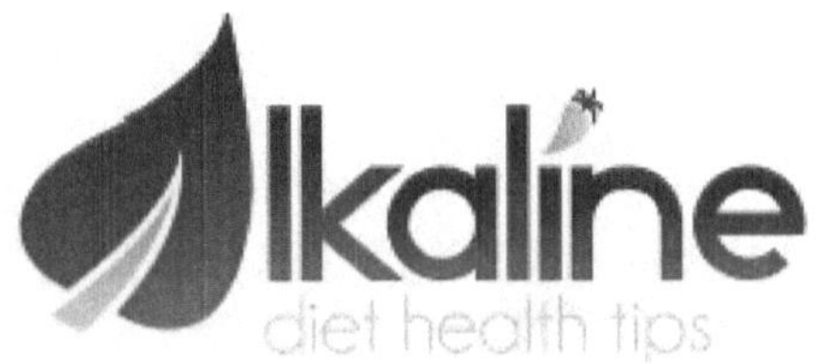

Acid & Alkaline Foods List

Alkaline Foods		Neutral / Moderately Acidic Foods		Very Acidic Foods	
Vegetables	Turnips	**Vegetables**	**Oils & Fats**	NOTE:	
Artichokes	Watercress	Black Olives	Sunflower Oil	ALL processed,	
Asparagus	Wheatgrass	Mushrooms	Avocado Oil	pre-packaged,	
Bamboo Shoots	Wild Greens		Coconut Oil	preserved, long-	
Broccoli	Dandelion Root	**Fruits**	Flax Oil	shelf life,	
Beetroots	Zucchini/Courgette	Fresh fruits are	Hemp Seed Oil	refined,	
Bell Peppers		alkaline but	Olive Oil	microwavable,	
Brussels Sprouts	**Fruits**	need to be	Saffower Oil	takeaway, fast,	
Cabbages	Avocados	eaten on their	Sesame Oil	dried, tinned,	
Carrots	Grapefruits	own or at least		meat, dairy &	
Cauliflowers	Lemons	first before any	(Use refined oils	frozen foods are	
Celery	Limes	other food. If	in VERY small	ACIDIC – such	
Chard	Tomatoes	combined with	quantities, or not	as cakes, chips,	
Chayote	(all above are most	fats and	at all)	burgers, tinned	
Chicory	alkaline fruits)	proteins, they		soup, granola	
Chives	Acai Berry	ferment,		bars, chocolate	
Collard Greens	Apples	causing		bars, pasta, ice	
Cucumbers	Apricots	indigestion and		cream & bread	
Dandelions	Bananas	acidity.			
Dills	Berries			**Vegetables**	
Eggplant	Cherries	Dried Fruits –		Pickled, Frozen &	
Endives	Coconuts	raisins, prunes,		Canned	
Garlic	Cranberries	apricots		Vegetables	
Green Beans	Currants				
Green Olives	Dates	Stewed Fruits		**Fruits**	
Green Peas	Figs			Tinned, sugared	
Greens (leafy)	Goji Berries			fruits	
Horseradishes	Gooseberries				
Kale	Grapes			**Oils & Fats**	
Kelp	Mangos			All Cooked,	
Leeks	Melons			Processed or	
Lettuces	Nectarines			Fried Oils,	
Mustard Greens	Oranges			Saturated Animal	
Okra	Papayas			Fats,	
Onions	Peaches			Hydrogenated &	
Oyster plants	Pears			Trans Fats	
Parsley	Pineapples				
Parsnips	Plums			**Grasses &**	
Peas (fresh)	Pomegranates			**Sprouts**	
Potatoes	Prunes			All Sprouts Are	
Radishes	Raisins			Alkaline	
Rutabagas	Raspberries				
Sea Veggies	Rhubarb				
Spinach	Other Tropical fruits –				
Sprouts (all)	e.g Durian, Jackfruit,				
Squash	Rambutan, Lychees,				
Sweet Potatoes	Mangosteen, Egg				
Sweetcorn	Fruit, Snake Fruit				

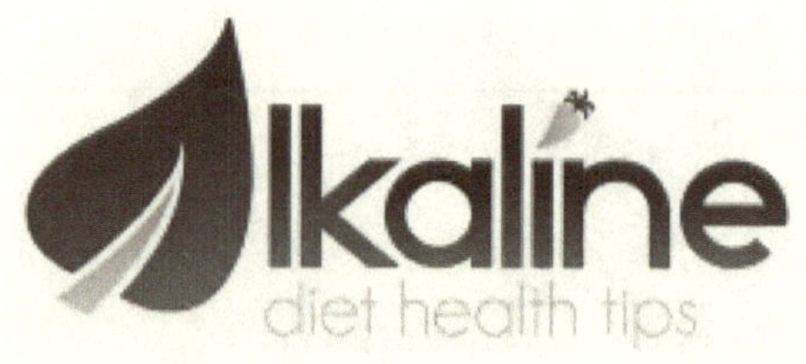

Alkaline Foods		Neutral / Moderately Acidic Foods		Acidic Foods	
Grains, Cereals & Breads Amaranth Buckwheat Kamut Millet Quinoa Spelt Sprouted Breads Sprouted Tortillas Yeast-Free Breads Dehydrated flax seed crackers **Sweets & Desserts** None **Beans & Legumes** All moderately acidic **Drinks** Alkaline Water Barley Grass Juice Coconut Water Fresh Lemon & Lime Water Fresh Veg Juices Green Drinks Green Tea Herbal Tea Wheatgrass Juice	**Diary & Meat** None **Condiments & Spices** (Unfermented Soy) Almond Butter Bee Pollen Bragg Aminos Chili Pepper Cinnamon Curry Powders Ginger Guacamole (fresh made) Herbs (all) Houmous Lemon Juice Lime Juice Sea Salt Spices (most) **Oriental Vegetables** Daikon Kombu Maitake Nori Reishi Sea Vegetables Shitake Umeboshi Wakame	**Grains, Cereals & Breads** Brown Rice Bulgar Wheat Home Made / Minimally Processed Breads Oats Wholegrain Pasta **Sweets & Desserts** Agave Honey Lo Han Guo Stevia **Beans & Legumes** Black Beans Canned Beans (Chick Peas) Garbanzo Beans Kidney Beans Lentils Lima Beans Mung Beans Navy Beans Pinto Beans Red Beans Soy Beans White Beans **Nuts & Seeds** Almond Butter Almonds Brazil Nuts Carraway Seeds Cashews Cumin Seeds Fennel Seeds Hazel Nuts Hemp Seeds Peanuts Pumpkin Seeds Sesame Seeds Sunflower Seeds Walnuts **Drinks** Tap, Bottled,	Carbonated & Unfiltered Water Pasteurised Fruit & Tomato Juice Kombucha Tea **Diary & Meat** Quorn (meat substitute) Tofu Whey (Raw) Yogurt (Organic Fresh) **Condiments & Spices** Apple Cider Vinegar Miso Tahini Spices (hot)	**Grains, Cereals & Breads** Barley Bran, oat Bran, wheat Bread Corn Corn Chips Cornstarch Crackers Flour Granola Noodles Pasta Processed Grains Rice Cakes Rye Spaghetti Wheat Germ White Rice Wheat Cous Cous **Sweets & Desserts** ALL Sugar, Sugar Products & Artificial Sweeteners **Beans & Legumes** All moderately acidic **Nuts & Seeds** All salted are moderately acidic	**Drinks** Alcohol Black Tea Cocoa Coffee Energy Drinks Milk Soda **Dairy & Meat** ALL products – including chicken, beef, pork, lamb, fish, cheese, milk, yoghurt, eggs **Condiments & Spices** Fermented Sauces Jams & Preserves Mayonnaise Soy Sauce Sweet Chilli Sauce Tomato Ketchup Vinegar

What Should We Eat; How Much; How Often?

The Bible mentions one of the sweeteners that we should use. This is honey; even the honeycomb may be eaten:

> *"My child, eat honey, for it is good, and the honeycomb is sweet to the taste."* Proverbs 24:13.

We should, however, eat it in moderation:

> *"Hast thou found honey? Eat so much as is sufficient for thee, lest thou be filled therewith, and vomit it... It is not good to eat too much honey..." Proverbs 25:16, 27 (NLT)*

Dates, which are also mentioned in the Bible, can also be used as a sweetener instead of sugar or honey.

Sweets, in excess, are not beneficial, as is evidenced by the increasing numbers of obesity and diabetes statistics. The American Heart Association (AHA) reports that our risk for diabetes and heart disease increases with these sugar-related abnormalities:

- obesity
- high blood pressure
- elevated blood triglycerides
- inflammation

Our intake of sugar has increased drastically. The American Heart Association (AHA) reported from its surveys, that the average human being consumes about 22.2 teaspoons of sugar per day. According to Dr. Bernard Jensen, "diabetes was being produced in animals, at will, in various universities and experimental hospitals, by feeding them too many starches and sugars. High blood pressure was produced by giving too much coffee to animals, and even cancer was caused in animals by using of certain coal tar drugs."

Coal tar dyes are synthetic products, once derived from coal tar but which are currently derived from petroleum sources. Coal tar dyes are used in foods, cosmetics and personal care products, such as hair dyes, shampoos and deodorants, over-the-counter and prescription drugs, and textiles. (*Chemical Encyclopedia*) Coal tar is a major ingredient in the production of food dyes and other additives, many of which are used in children's cereals.

CHAPTER **4**

GLUTTONY

"Gluttony is lust of the mind," said Thomas Hobbes. The twenty-third chapter of the book of Proverbs exhorts us to *"put a knife to our throat if we are given to appetite."* *(23:2)* Solomon later warns, in the same chapter, that *"the drunkard and glutton shall come to poverty."* (verse 21)

A glutton is a person who eats and drinks excessively or voraciously; a person with a remarkably great desire or capacity for something.

There is much to be said for the biblical way of eating. God gave clear commands. The 'how much' has also been addressed, the emphasis being on moderation. Before great success and disregard of God's Word came into being; before creamy sauces and sugar-filled nutrient-empty but addictive foods, the Bible shows that in the earlier years, the children of Israel ate twice per day.

After their exodus from Egypt, while in the wilderness, they received meat (quails) from God in the evening. In the morning, he gave them food, which they called manna. They ate manna for forty years in the wilderness and suffered no diseases or vitamin or mineral deficiencies during that time. That's good manna! Moses, the Scriptures tell us, was in excellent health; he was 120 years old before the time of his death, yet *"his eye was not dim, nor his natural force abated." Deuteronomy 34:7*

"Happy is the land whose king is a noble leader and whose leaders feast at the proper time to gain strength for their work, not to get drunk." (NLT)

History shows that most nations of the earlier centuries ate twice per day, with the first meal being very light and occurring between 11:00 and noon. Some peoples ate only one big meal, with a piece of fruit (figs for some), at or close to noon. Nomadic and hunting tribes seemed to eat closer to noon, after having returned from hunting. If their hunt was unfruitful, they did not eat that first meal. In a sense, those tribes practiced what we now call intermittent fasting.

Dr. Herbert Shelton, author of *The Hygienic System Orthotrophy* wrote about these eating habits of earlier nations and noted that the Greco and Roman empires tended to eat in this manner as well. In England, the practice was the same for many centuries. It was only in more modern times that the rich, as an indication of success, began to eat more often and more richly. (*The Hygienic System Orthotrophy*, Dr. Herbert M. Shelton, 1935)

A Little Wine

Wine was used for celebrations and for medicinal purposes. The Lord Jesus, at the marriage in Cana, was asked to help because the wine was finished. There, He performed his first miracle on the earth by turning water into wine. Had the drinking of wine been improper or unlawful, his mother would not have asked him to help. The apostle Paul also advised Timothy,

> *"Use a little wine for thy stomach's sake and thine often infirmities."* 1 Timothy 5:23.

There is a correct use of wine. Notice, in his exhortation

to Timothy, that the apostle Paul said, *"a little wine."* Wine may be drunken but in moderation.

"Do not carouse with drunkards or feast with gluttons, for they are on their way to poverty, and too much sleep clothes them in rags. Proverbs 23:20-21 NLT

Wine is a mocker, strong drink a brawler, and whoever is led astray by it is not wise. Proverbs 20:1 ESV

Drunkenness was not encouraged, then or now. Whenever there was a situation of imbibing to excess, there were always dire consequences. Think of Noah, Lot, and Nabal.

The Bible explains the destruction that wine in excess can bring. Wine mocks those who profess to be able to control themselves. Wine betrays, if given the slightest leeway. Mixed wine speaks to the additives that are now combined with the fruit of the vine, the stronger alcohols that wreak so much havoc on a system that was not designed to cool its fire.

"Who has woe? Who has sorrow? Who has strife? Who has complaining? Who has wounds without cause? Who has redness of eyes? Those who tarry long over wine; those who go

to try mixed wine. Do not look at wine when it is red, when it sparkles in the cup and goes down smoothly. In the end it bites like a serpent and stings like an adder. Your eyes will see strange things, and your heart utter perverse things. ..." Proverbs 23:29-35 ESV

"Moreover, wine is a traitor, an arrogant man who is never at rest. His greed is as wide as Sheol (the grave); like death, he has never enough. He gathers for himself all nations and collects as his own all peoples." Habakkuk 2:5 ESV

"Woe to those who rise early in the morning, that they may run after strong drink, who tarry late into the evening as wine inflames them!" Isaiah 5:11 ESV

God, in His great wisdom and love for His people, saw the propensity of man to experiment; therefore, he warned them repeatedly.

A Little Sleep

Sleep, our much-needed resource, can also be excessive. Research shows a connection between too much sleep and too little energy. Too much appears to upset the body's rhythms and increase daytime fatigue.

"Love not sleep, lest you come to poverty; open your eyes, and you shall be satisfied with bread." Proverbs 20:13 KJV

"…But you, lazybones, how long will you sleep? When will you wake up?

A little extra sleep, a little more slumber, a little folding of the hands to rest— then poverty will pounce on you like a bandit; scarcity will attack you like an armed robber." Proverbs 6:9-10 NLT

The Right Kind of Food

The children of Israel, because of disobedience, were captured by the Babylonians. Their captor, King Nebuchadnezzar, chose from among them some boys whom he wanted to train and teach the tongue of the Chaldeans (Babylonianians). He wanted boys who were "gifted in all wisdom, possessing knowledge, and quick to understand." Among the boys whom he chose were Daniel, Hananiah, Mishael, and Azariah. These boys were between 11-13 years old.

The king wanted these boys to be fed with the king's

meat and wine for a period of three years, at which they would begin to stand before the king in service. Daniel decided that he did not wish to eat in this manner and asked the eunuch who was given the king's order to allow him and his three friends to eat in the Hebrew manner for ten days. Then, if they appeared worse than the other boys who were eating the king's meat, the eunuch could then deal with them as he saw fit.

Daniel's decision made the overseeing eunuch fearful because he had his orders. Perhaps, he, like so many others, had subscribed to the belief that a plant-based diet would make the four boys look poorly and ultimately, worse-looking than the other boys who were consuming the king's meat and wine. Sadly, that is the very thought that many people entertain today.

Daniel and his three Hebrew friends proceeded to eat pulse and water, a diet with which they were familiar. Several websites, inclusive of restorehealth.org, explain that the original word for pulse is *zeroa*, which is defined as vegetables, such as lentils, chickpeas, or some other form of grain. "*Zara*, the root word for *zeroa*, is found in the context of that which God gave to mankind to eat at creation.

The definition for vegetable enlarges considerably when God defines food. The word *zara*, according to the Enhanced Strong's Lexicon means to sow or scatter seed. This indicates the plants' ability to make seeds that are able to produce yet another plant." [Klondike Mountain Health Retreat, www.retreat2restorehealth.orf/daniel-pulsehtml].

Some examples of these 'seed scatterers' are potatoes, garlic, beets, carrots, onions, walnuts, almonds, sunflower seeds, and cashew nuts.

"At the end of ten days, the four boys' "countenances appeared fairer and fatter in flesh than all the children which did eat the portion of the king's meat." (Daniel 1:15)

Was there something wrong with the king's meat? One can only speculate, since no reason was proffered. Vegetables do provide a significant boost to the body, more so, because they are more easily assimilated into the system. Vegetables are rich in nutrients; this, the children of Israel knew. May we truly learn this as well.

It is determined by some that God's explicit instructions were given not only to show the special separation of the children of Israel from the other nations, but that their observance of the "Kashrut cultivates self-control and discipline and encourages mindful eating." [Source: "Anonymous. "Keeping Kosher: Jewish Dietary Laws." ReligionFacts. February 8, 2007. [Accessed August 2, 2012] (http://www.religionfacts.com/judaisim/practices/kosher.htm) .

Our progressive world has rationalized away many of God's instructions, deeming them outdated or applicable only to the children of Israel. Some even determine that those rules applied only under the dispensation of law. Regardless of our rationalizations, we are unable to dispute the consequences of our disdain. Illness has run rampant throughout the centuries, and while medical knowledge has helped to lengthen lives, the side effects from some medications and surgical procedures are alarming.

A much more simple solution to healthy living would be to adhere to godly instruction. A car manufacturer provides a manual for his model, even detailing the type of gasoline that will enable optimum performance. He even advises on the type of cleaner to be used and recommends oil changes and maintenance at regular intervals. Many of us adhere to these instructions because we want our vehicles to last for a long time. We fear having a break-down at an inopportune time, and we love a shiny vehicle that looks 'like new' while it is ours. Ought we not, then, to try to not care for our bodies with even one-half that level of attention?

Chapter 5

A Land with Wheat and Barley

~Uses of plants and herbs~

"For the Lord your God is bringing you into a good land… a land with wheat and barley, vines and fig trees, pomegranates, olive oil, and honey…" Deuteronomy 8:7-8

When God prepared the land of Canaan for the Israelites, He filled it with the best of foods – foods that nourished and which could also be replanted and cultivated, providing not only food for mankind and animals, but also means of honest labor and sources of income and trade.

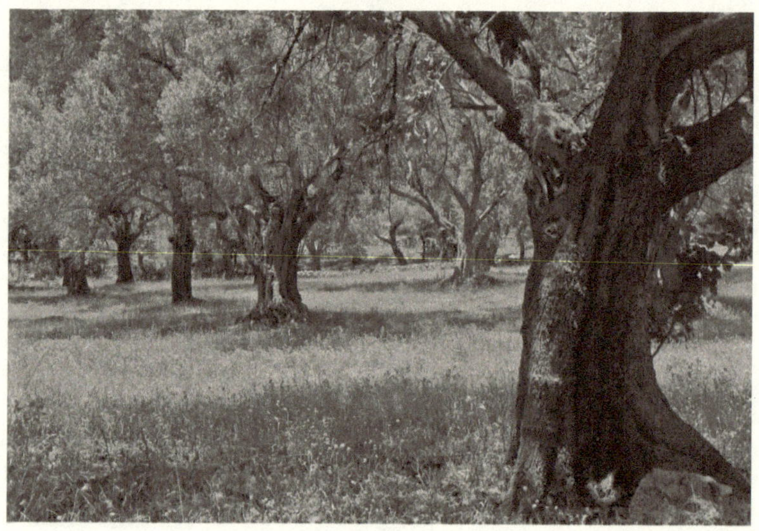

Olive trees

Olives: In ancient times, olive oil was used to cook, to light lamps, and as soap and skin conditioner. The fragrant oils were rubbed into the skin. Today, the olive remains a popular food and its golden oil is a coveted commodity. Moreover, olive oil has become more popular since the discovery that it lowers cholesterol and aids in cardiovascular health. Olive oil is alkaline and is also now known to contain anti-cancer properties.

Grapes: In ancient times, grapes were used for seasoning and in vinegars. The wine that is pressed from them was used in celebrations and blessings.

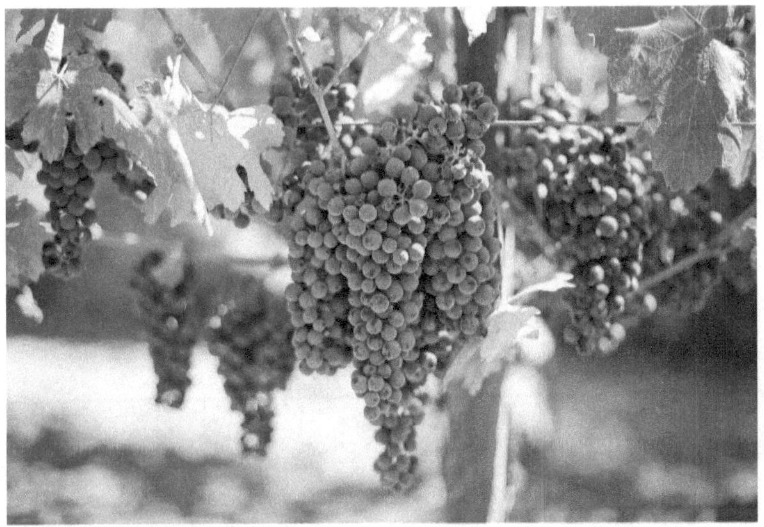

Grapes of Napa Valley

Research now shows their numerous health benefits; (though not seedless grapes, for much benefit is in the seeds). Grapes provide phytonutrients, mainly phenols, and polyphenols, and contain important vitamins such as vitamins B6, K, A, and C. They are rich in antioxidants. Flavonoids, like myricetin and quercetin, in grapes help the body to reduce the damage caused by free radicals and slow aging. Because grapes, especially dark grapes, are rich in iron, the fruit is recommended to ward off heart disease.

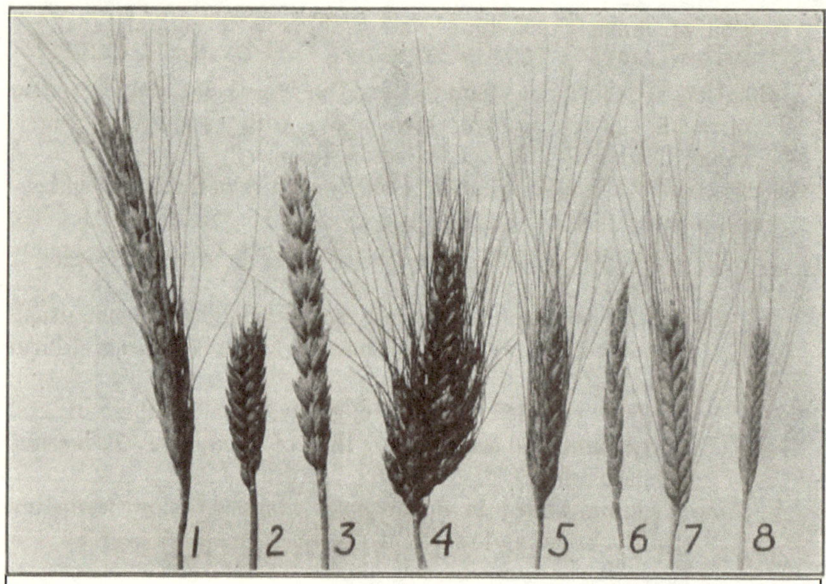

Illustration of different types of wheat: (1) Polish wheat (2) Club wheat (3) Common bread wheat (4) Poulard wheat (5) Durum wheat (6) Spelt (7) Emmer (8) Einkorn.

The Library of Congress/Flickr The Commons

Wheat: The wheat of modern times is not the wheat of the Bible. Most of today's wheat was crafted, a dwarf-wheat that was developed around 1960 by cross-breeding and genetic manipulation.

Einkorn is the most ancient wheat, offering essential dietary and trace minerals. It's a good source of protein, iron, dietary fiber, thiamine and a number of other B-vitamins. It also contains a significant amount of the powerful antioxidant, lutein, with higher antioxidant levels than durum wheat. It has nutrients, whereas modern wheat, which was created in a lab, does not.

Emmer is said to be the grain of the ancient Mesopotamians. It is also known as *farro* and has many beneficial and healthy proteins.

Kamut is another ancient relative of wheat and is supposedly of Egyptian heritage. Because it, like the others, has not been cross-bred, it is more easy for many people to digest. Kamut is also high in protein.

Barley: In the biblical times, barley was the poor-man's

staple - eaten as porridge and made into barley cakes. Cattle and other livestock were also fed barley. Today, 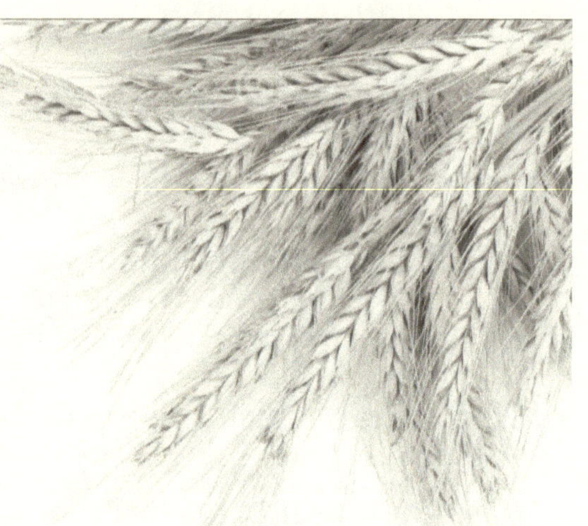 the grain has become a marginal culinary ingredient used in soups and stews.

The dietary fiber in barley serves as food for the friendly bacteria in the large intestine, producing the fatty acid, butyric acid, which helps maintain a healthy colon and providing fuel to its cells. Barley contains the eight essential amino acids, making it a complete protein in our diet.

Figs: The fig tree — with its distinctive leaves - used as

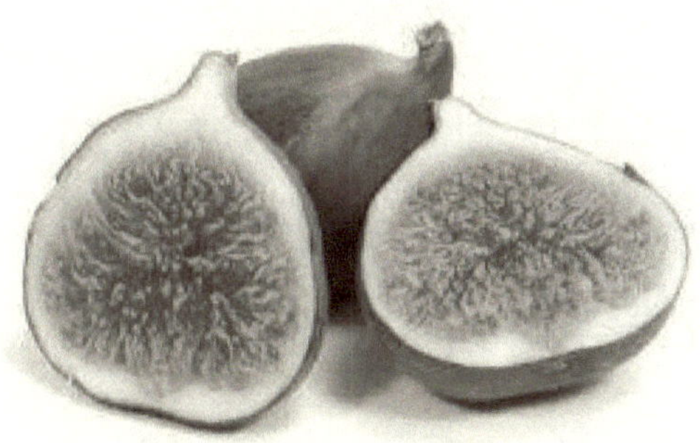

clothes by Adam and Eve - is a ubiquitous part of the Israeli landscape. In biblical times the fig was eaten fresh or as a seasoning, in addition to being used to make honey and alcohol.

The sweet, chewy fruit is rich in antioxidants and claims its place in traditional medicine. It is used dried, whole, ground or in paste form to fight several diseases. When King Hezekiah was dying of boils, Isaiah instructed the king's men to "take a lump of figs and lay it on the boils, and King Hezekiah recovered.

Dates: Date palms are found in the hotter inland rift valley. In biblical times they grew in the Jordan Valley, but with modern irrigation

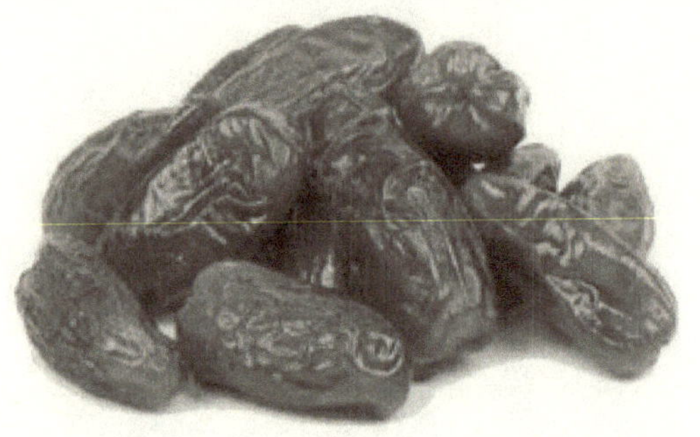

techniques, the palms have also taken root near the Dead Sea and further south in the Arava. In the biblical era dates were made into honey, and many believe the notion of the "land flowing with milk and honey" actually referred to date honey.

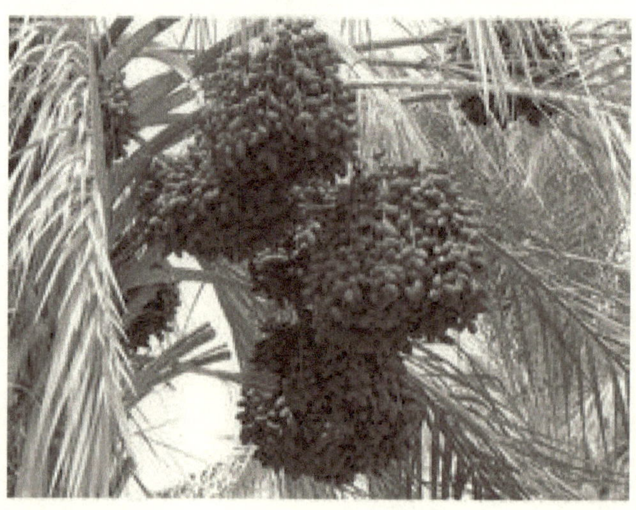

A date palm tree

Dates are quite rich in vitamins B6, A, and K which support bone development and eye health. They are said to have the following benefits:

• Promote digestive health and relieving constipation

• Boosting heart health

• Anti-Inflammatory (high magnesium levels)

• Reduce blood pressure – (magnesium and potassium)

• Reduced Stroke Risk (magnesium)

• Healthy Pregnancy and Delivery

• Boosting Brain Health (vitamin B6 levels)

Source: http://naturalsociety.com/health-benefits-of-dates-7-reasonseat-date-fruit/#ixzz57O91Y7Tp

Pomegranates: Pomegranate trees are prevalent in Israeli

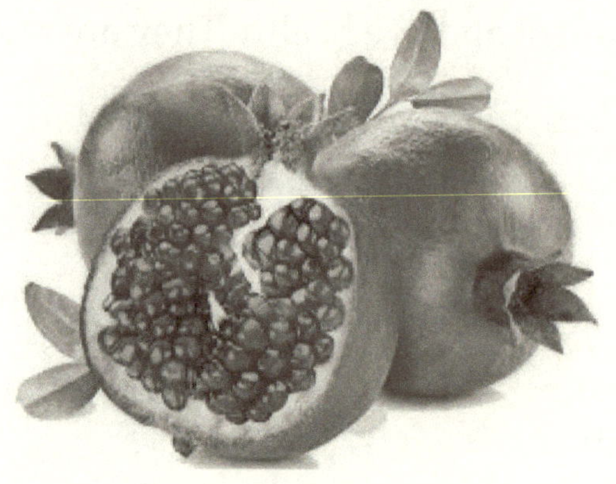 gardens. The tree with its rich green leaves and red flowers becomes heavy with fruit for Rosh Hashanah

(New Year). In biblical times the plump red fruit was used for making wine and seasonings in addition to its function as a dye. It was also appreciated for its aesthetic qualities, particularly the crown near the stem. Tradition has it that a pomegranate has 613 seeds to represent the 613 commandments in the Torah (the five books of Moses).

(Source: Jewish Virtual *Library*, American-Israeli Cooperative Enterprise)

EATING IN "DUE SEASON"

God speaks of eating our meals *"in due season"* (or the appropriate time) in Ecclesiastes 10:17. He stated that we are blessed when we eat for strength, rather than for drunkenness (excess).

In our world, we are encouraged to eat at least six meals per day. For some of us, unfortunately, this type of grazing pattern is unnecessary. The quality of work that some of us are required to do is not to such a strenuous extent that our energy is so quickly burnt. In addition, sometimes, the food in our stomachs has not even been digested before another meal comes traveling down the digestive tract. Sometimes, the reason for waning energy during the day is improper nutrition.

This constant eating cycle puts our system under pressure to digest without ceasing. Because of the constant work of the body's organs become stressed; the liver and other eliminative organs do not have a chance to sufficiently divest the body of harmful toxins.

With all of our medical advancement, the incidence of organ stress and failure is increasing quite alarmingly. "In the United States, for example, the number of patients on the waiting list [for organ transplants due to organ failure] in the year 2006 had risen to over 95,000, while the number of patient deaths was over 6,300 [because of organ failure]". (US National Library of Medicine, National Institutes of Health)

Our purpose, where food is concerned, should be to eat to live, rather than live to eat. Allowing the body time to digest food is essential.

FASTING

An effective method of eating to live is by occasional fasting. Fasting, by definition is voluntarily refraining from food for varying lengths of time and is also used as a medical therapy for many conditions. Fasting is used as a spiritual practice in many religions (The Free Medical Dictionary). It is used for both spiritual and physical health. Fasting cleans the body internally. Depending upon the type of fast in observance (there are three types), herbs were sometimes used in the cleansing process.

The three types of fast are as follow:

6. The Normal Fast which involved the total abstinence of food but not water. *"Jesus did eat nothing." Luke 4:2*

7. The Absolute Fast which seemed to have lasted no longer than three days because it is a total abstinence from food and water. Saul *"neither did eat nor drink." Acts 9:9*

8. The Partial Fast where the emphasis seems to be on restriction in diet, rather than total abstinence. *"I ate no delicacies, no meat or wine entered my mouth, nor did I anoint myself at all, for the full three weeks." Daniel 10:3*

[Source: Fausset's Bible Dictionary]

"William A. Lane, addressing the Johns Hopkins Hospital and Medical College said: 'Gentlemen, I will never die of cancer. I am taking measures to prevent it… It is caused by poisons created in our bodies by the food we eat… What we should do, then, if we would avoid cancer, is to eat… raw fruits and vegetables; first, that we may be better nourished; secondly, that we may more easily eliminate waste products… We have been studying germs when we should have been studying diet and drainage. The world has been on the wrong track. The answer has been within ourselves all the time… Drain the body of its poisons, feed it properly, and the miracle is done. Nobody need have cancer who will take the trouble to avoid it.' Lane lived to be 87 years old and died in an auto accident during the Second World War in London." (from Why Christians Get Sick by Rev. George Malkmus)

THREE PRINCIPLES OF CURE

Dr. Bernard Jensen in his book "*The Science and Practice of Iridology*, wrote,

"There are three principles of cure which we should particularly remember. First, the body must have a healthy blood stream, for without this, the body cannot have a healthy cell structure. Since cell life is dependent upon the blood, this must be kept clean and toxin-free… "

"The second principle is very important. It is that the blood must circulate rapidly enough to supply cell structures with all the necessary building elements. It must circulate fast enough to give the body the opportunity to build and repair as rapidly as is required."

The third principle is rest. Rest cures… Rest allows the body to recuperate and regenerate. Tiredness was given to us as a barometer and fatigue is the first symptom of all disease." (p.43.

The Science and Practice of Iridology.)

CHAPTER 6

HEALTH EXPLORED: CLEAN BODY

In God's eyes, it was not enough to ensure that the inside of the body is clean; there are standards for the outside as well. History has taught us that for many years, people died from unsanitary surgical procedures. In the 1800s, more than 25000 pregnant women and new mothers died in the United States at the unwashed hands of doctors.

It was even worse in Europe. The famous Allegemeine Krakenhaus hospital in Vienna, for example, developed quite a reputation because one of every six women on its maternity ward died. They were taken into the autopsy room and autopsies were performed on them the next morning. The practice of the doctors and medical students was to perform the autopsies first thing in the morning, then go to perform their rounds on the medical wards – without washing their hands! The death toll was staggering.

Mary Wollstonecraft, a well-known Anglo-Irish feminist and writer of the 1700s, died ten days after giving birth to her daughter, Mary Shelley, because her doctor touched her uterus with hands that had been pricked by an autopsy tool. The medical profession, of all people, should know that dead bodies carry bacteria, are harbingers of disease, and are extremely toxic.

When a young doctor, Ignaz Semmelweis, noticed the high death numbers, specifically among women, he instituted a rule in his ward, that every physician must wash his hands before examining the living. The death numbers dropped significantly thereafter, from fifty-seven women dying in April 1847 on Semmelweis's ward before the law, to one in forty-two women only two months thereafter. By July, the rate of death was one in eighty-four women. Semmelweis' theory was treated with disdain by the medical profession and the deaths on other wards and in other hospitals continued.

The book of Leviticus provides detailed records of God telling his people how to clean themselves after contact with anything that was dead or diseased. In some instances of contact, the defiled person was considered "unclean until the even" (chapter 11 verse 32) and had to remain separate from the people until then, and, even then, only after he had carefully cleansed himself.

Some issues of uncleanness required seven days of separation from the people. God foresaw the potential for disease and death, and took care to instruct his people on the safest cleaning practices. God even specified that the washing of hands and bathing of flesh should not merely be in a basin of standing water but rather, in running water. This is something that has only begun to be emphasized in modern times.

The children of Israel, throughout their generations, use high heat when washing dishes or laundry. Some eating utensils are soaked for several days before washing, especially if dairy and meat are consumed. [Sources: Jewish Virtual Library – Kashrut: Jewish Dietary Laws. {www.jewishvirtual… 2012 The American-Israeli Cooperative Enterprise}]

God gave instructions concerning diseases of the skin and eruptions, even so far as menstruation and bodily fluids that resulted from sexual intercourse. The act of cleanliness went even further; He instructed the children of Israel in the practice of circumcision. Once again, the reason might not have seemed readily apparent to the listener, but does God really need to explain himself to anyone?

A WOMAN'S TIME

We reap the consequences of our defiance. God, in his directives to Moses, gave the following instruction:

"…you shall not approach a woman to uncover her nakedness as long as she is in her customary impurity." Leviticus 15:19

Simply put: don't have sexual relations while a woman is menstruating. The blood contains waste that is the breakdown of an unfertilized egg. According to the NIH, a woman's menstrual cycle causes an overgrowth of the bacteria called *Staphylococcus aureus*. During intercourse, a male may become infected with these bacteria.

[Source: Toxic Shock Syndrome - How To Information | eHow.com http://www.ehow.com/toxic-shock-syndrome/#ixzz26fomZ5bD]

ON CIRCUMCISION

"He who is eight days old among you shall be circumcised…" Genesis 17:12

God decreed a specific time in a male baby's life because the body's natural supply of vitamin K which aids in blood clotting, is not present during the first three days of a child's life. As a child begins to nurse, vitamin K begins to develop. At day five, there is a low level. "After five to seven days of breast-feeding, infants have built up enough vitamin K to allow blood clotting to withstand circumstances." (Russell, *What the* Bible Says About Healthy Living – p.11)

Dr. Rex Russell recounted an incident that occurred at the beginning of his surgical practice. He stated that his first case was a newborn male who was circumcised on day three of his life. Dr. Russell stated that it was routine procedure to circumcise babies during the first three days of their lives. After completing the circumcision, he noticed that the patient's bandage was soaked with blood four hours after the procedure. He administered vitamin K to aid in clotting the blood but the bleeding did not stop completely until several days later. Russell noted that the child had begun life with a needless risk.

The U.S. National Library of Medicine reported that "a newborn boy is usually circumcised before he leaves the hospital. Jewish boys, however, are circumcised when they are eight days old… There is no compelling medical rationale for the procedure in healthy boys…" (Medline Plus. Maryland: 2012. www.nlm.nih.gov/medlineplus/news)

The international Coalition for Genital Integrity stated that Thymos: Journal of Boyhood Studies estimates that more than 100 baby boys die from circumcision complications in the United States each year. (www.icgi.org)

In more recent years, it has become obvious why the cutting of the foreskin is so essential. In most cases where there is no circumcision of the penis, it is difficult to clean beneath the folds of skin, especially as it is usually tight and unretractable. As such, bacteria tend to build beneath the foreskin. Smegma bacillus, the bacteria that produce cancer can grow there.

During sexual intercourse, bacteria are deposited at the cervix of the uterus. If the membrane of the uterus is intact, little harm results. If lacerations exist, as they do after childbirth and in one or two other situations, then irritation develops. Where there is much irritation, the chance of cancer increases because of bacteria; and it makes sense then, that cervical cancer is high in women who have had children, and whose mates are not circumcised. There is also the possibility of cancer of the penis from bacteria.

The problem of uncleanness in medical practice still exists, though not to the devastating degree that it did in the earlier centuries. The Baltimore Sun published an article in 2007 which reported that pregnancy for poor, women in early 19th century Vienna was "lethal," because of unsanitary habits by doctors. ABC News' Chris Kilmer reported in 2009 that the hand washing rate is low among doctors. Kilmer included an article by two New York Times' writers, Stephen J. Dunbar and Steven D. Levitt. The article, titled Selling Soap, made the following observation:

"It may seem a mystery why doctors, of all people, practice poor hand hygiene. But as Bender huddled with the hospital's leadership, they identified a number of reasons. For starters, doctors are very busy. And a sink isn't always handy.... There also seem to be psychological reasons for noncompliance. The first is what might be called a perception deficit. In one Australian medical study, doctors self-reported their hand-washing rate at 73 percent, whereas when these same doctors were observed, their actual rate was a paltry 9 percent. The second psychological reason, according to one Cedars-Sinai doctor, is arrogance...."

Source: ABCNews.go.com]

"...if thou wilt indeed hear the voice of the LORD thy God, and do things pleasing before him, and will hearken to his commands, and keep all his ordinances, no disease...shall I bring upon thee, for I am the LORD thy God that heals thee." Exodus 15:26

OFFENSES AGAINST THE BODY

"For God is not the author of confusion, but of peace..." 1 Corinthians 14:33 KJV

Whatever God says is clearly stated and no interpretation is required. It is not His intent to be misunderstood by His people. There is therefore, no need for an interpreter when He states that sexual sin brings great harm to the body. It brings harm on many levels: physically, spiritually, morally, and emotionally.

"Flee from sexual immorality. All other sins a man commits are outside his body, but he who sins

sexually sins against his own body..."
1 Corinthians 6:18

The havoc that sexual sin wreaks is often quite painful and devastating. The eye takes a picture that is forever imprinted upon the mind. Sexual sin affects the individual as well as the partner with whom the sin is committed. It matters not if the act was committed when the individual was single. The experience can become an albatross, the Bible has shown:

"Can a man scoop fire into his lap without his clothes being burned? Can a man walk on hot coals without his feet being scorched? So is he who sleeps with another man's wife; no one who touches her will go unpunished." Proverbs 6:27-29

God's standards for sexual conduct are essential for life and good health. The introduction of AIDS and other sexually transmitted diseases (STDs) is testament to a refusal to adhere to instructions. Unfortunately, children suffer for these sexual sins, as well, since the HIV virus is passed through the birth canal to the birthing baby. The Centers for Disease Control reports that there are approximately 19 million new STD infections each year, and almost one-half of them are occurring among young people between 15 and 24. Teen-age girls have the highest rates of gonorrhea in the nation and teen-age boys are second.

Promiscuity, whether in heterosexual or homosexual relationships, in addition to being against God's laws, also causes increase in diseases. Statistics in the 1990's showed that if one has an STD, his chances of getting AIDS from an infected partner increases 100 times.

According to healthpeople.gov, 43% of homosexuals say that they have had 500 or more sexual partners in their lifetime. Only 1% of homosexuals say they have had four or less sexual partners in their lifetime. As one person puts it, the Bible, in no way, condemns filial love between people of the same sex, but it does state that *sexual conduct* between those people is sin.

Sexual sin *does* defile us and causes us harm - harm to our is emotional, physical, psychological and, yes, spiritual health. God provided laws for our health, growth, and overall well-being. [Source: www.Healthypeople.gov. Accessed September 9, 2012.]

In our "whatever goes" world, it is becoming more easy to ignore the words of the Bible, especially as it applies to sexual immorality, and do that which feels good. Disobedience has a price, however, chief of which are heartbreak, distrust, diseases and death. Fornication breeds distrust in whoever practices it. Adultery has its own set of woes, including distrust, hurt, and fear. We are over-run with sexually-transmitted diseases, among them gonorrhea, the Human Papilloma Virus (HPV) and Acquired Immune Deficiency Syndrome (AIDS). Promiscuity is the main cause of the spread of these diseases. The apostle Paul warned against close associations with those who see no problem with certain lifestyles:

> *"But now I am writing to you not to associate with anyone who bears the name of brother if he is guilty of sexual immorality or greed, or is an idolater, reviler, drunkard, or swindler—not even to eat with such a one."* 1 Corinthians 5:11 ESV

> *Do not be misled: "Bad company corrupts good character." 1 Corinthians 15:33*

> *"Don't you realize that this sin is like a little yeast that spreads through the whole batch of dough? Get rid of the old "yeast" by removing this wicked person from among you. Then you will be like a fresh batch of dough made without yeast..."* 1 Corinthians 5:6 NLT

An article by the Los Angeles Times entitled *Parents' Affairs Can Devastate Kids* stated thus: "When parents go outside the marital vows, they are taking a shotgun and firing into a crowd. That shot will hurt a spouse, sure, but most likely, it will also take out some people who were never intended to get hit."

Chapter 7

Financial Health

Work is an integral part of man's constitution; it has been since the beginning of creation. Although he lived in an amply-stocked garden with every possible fruit, vegetable and herb for his delight, Adam had a job. He named the animals when God brought them to him, and he tended the garden.

Although sin had not yet entered the garden, God did not create Adam to sit idly. Later, after his sin and banishment from the garden, Adam still had to work, except that he had to sweat to obtain his bread. Adam was expected to work, as are we. Indeed, the apostle Paul reminded the church at Corinth that

"… The Scriptures tell us that if any would not work, neither should he eat." *2 Thessalonians 2:10*

There are Scriptures that provide step-by-step instructions with regard to our day to day existence:

"The plan of the diligent lead surely to plenty, but those of everyone who is hasty, surely to poverty." *Proverbs 13:11*

Know the state of your finances. Do not live with financial blinders but rather, know how much you have, how much you can spend, and make provision to set resources aside for emergencies and lean times.

"Be thou diligent to know the state of thy flocks, and look well to thy herbs." *Proverbs 27:23*

Laziness does not profit, nor will it fill your stomach. Make every effort to find something to do, even if it does not match your dream job or task. We are exhorted to observe a tiny creature and take our cue from its dedication.

"Go to the ant, o sluggard, observe her ways and be

wise, which, having no chief, officer or ruler, prepares her food in the summer, and gathers her provision in the harvest." Proverbs 6:6-8

Honest labor, with a plan, is rewarding:

"Wealth gotten by vanity (dishonesty) shall be diminished: but he that gathers by labor shall increase." Proverbs 13:11

Honest labor should be exactly that. Anything less is a robber, both of the offender and the victim. In addition, we are cautioned on the manner in which we should behave, if we become successful.

Don't make your living by extortion or put your hope in stealing. And if your wealth increases, don't make it the center of your life. Psalm 62:10 NLT

Honest labor also allows one to sleep in peace:

"In peace I will both lie down and sleep; for you alone, O Lord, make me dwell in safety." Psalm 4:8

We are exhorted to use wisdom regarding our finances. Spending heedlessly without stewardship results in disaster and cultivates irresponsibility:

"The thoughts (plans) of the diligent tend only to plenteousness; but of every one that is hasty only to want." Proverbs 21:5 KJV

Careless spending results in debt which leads to borrowing and working even harder to fix the debt issue. This then causes stress, unhappiness and the thwarting of plans. The wisest man who ever lived told us that debt is a cruel master.

"The rich rules over the poor, and the borrower is servant to the lender." Proverbs 22:7

The apostle Paul, in his letter to the Romans, exhorted them to *"owe no man anything, but to love one another..." Romans 13:8*

THE ROAD TO MATERIAL HEALTH

King Solomon learned, much to his consternation, that while there is nothing wrong with beautiful things, there is futility in pursuing a lavish lifestyle, to the exclusion of everything else. He wrote:

"I also tried to find meaning by building huge homes for myself and by planting beautiful vineyards. ⁵ I made gardens and parks, filling them with all kinds of fruit trees. ⁶ I built reservoirs to collect the water to irrigate my many flourishing groves. ⁷ I bought slaves, both men and women, and others were born into my household. I also owned large herds and flocks, more than any of the kings who had lived in Jerusalem before me. ⁸ I collected great sums of silver and gold, the treasure of many kings and provinces. I hired wonderful singers, both men and women, and had many beautiful concubines. I had everything a man could desire!

⁹ So I became greater than all who had lived in Jerusalem before me, and my wisdom never failed me. ¹⁰ Anything I wanted, I would take. I denied myself no pleasure. I even found great pleasure in hard work, a reward for all my labors. [11] But as I looked at everything I had worked so hard to accomplish, it was all so meaningless—like chasing the wind. There was nothing really worthwhile anywhere. Ecclesiastes 2 New Living Translation (NLT).

If your sole purpose is to work to be rich, you will be rich in possessions but poor in spirit and decrepit in soul. We do not exist in isolation; live to help others and be a source of encouragement and help. Help need not be monetary, though if you have enough to give, then consider doing that. Ultimately, life is about waking each day and asking yourself, 'Whom can I help today?'

Someone may need a smile, a compliment, a friendly word, a hand to prevent him from falling or a hand to help him up, if he has. Life is realizing that you are a catalyst; your act of kindness may save someone's life, though you may never know it.

Chapter 8

Physical Principles – All Work and No Play

Consider a car that is left with its engine running incessantly. We all know what will happen after a time - burn-out. Parts will need to be replaced, fuel and other fluids will become depleted, and there will be overheating. Even inanimate objects need a break; how much more we?

The Bible deals with the whole man, providing clear instructions for every facet of the human existence. There is more to man than his spiritual self, even though he is a spiritual being. In addition to cleanliness, food and sexual morality, God gives clear instructions on building a healthy balance between work, physical activity, and rest.

Our society does not allow for rest. Beset by obligations and responsibilities, we are tired, restless, unfocused, irritable, depressed, overweight, and ill. God, in his wisdom, exhorted us to rest and he led by example. He worked for six days in the creation of the world, then rested on the seventh day. He did not rest because He was tired; no, He set this day apart, marking it sanctified (holy) for fellowship with His highest creation, Adam and Eve. [See *Genesis 2:2-3*].

> *"And he [Jesus] said to them, "Come away by yourselves to a desolate place and rest a while." For many were coming and going, and they had no leisure even to eat." Mark 6:31*

Following the divine demonstration, then, work comes first, and then rest. Both are optimal for health and wellbeing. Work is both physical and mental. It brings a sense of purpose, of accomplishment. After a period of engaging work, there needs to be rest. Why? Whenever energy is expended, waste accrues.

There is waste from the buildup of toxins, as your body works. We sweat, we expel extra air, and we use and wear out cells in the body as we expend energy. Your body needs time to slough off this waste. If it is not given the opportunity to do so, fatigue sets in because your body is now lugging around dead cells and toxins that it does need and cannot use. While it is carrying that waste, it is still working to perform all of its other functions.

There are other contributors to stress and fatigue in the body. Acidity leading to acidosis from insufficient hydration; poor dietary habits, insufficient exercise, and poor oxygenation head the list.

One might think that mental activity does not make one tired. This is far from true. Over time, prolonged mental activity causes stress to build. Your body yearns for a break. You rub your eyes; massage the back of your neck, sigh deeply, sometimes without realizing it, and your muscles begin to tighten. That brings more stress and fatigue. Productivity and performance then decrease. The physical muscles need stretching and rest to relax and the mind needs rest and sleep to recharge.

So many times, we ignore our need for rest or we coerce our body into pressing on by feeding it coffee or some other stimulant. Underneath the caffeine haze, though, the body is still giving signals that it needs rest. Fatigue builds, and the body requires more stimulants to keep up the façade.

King Solomon summed it in these words:

"It is useless for you to work so hard from early morning until late at night, anxiously working for food to eat; for God gives rest to his loved ones."
Psalm 127:2 NLT

God determined that even the animals should rest – it was that important to the quality of life:

"Six days thou shalt do thy work, and on the seventh day thou shalt rest: that thine ox and thine ass may rest, and the son of thy handmaid, and the stranger, may be refreshed. Exodus 23:12 (KJV)

King Solomon reflected on his life, the wisdom with which he was blessed, possessions he had acquired, and summarized:

[12] People who work hard sleep well, whether they eat little or much. But the rich seldom get a good night's sleep.

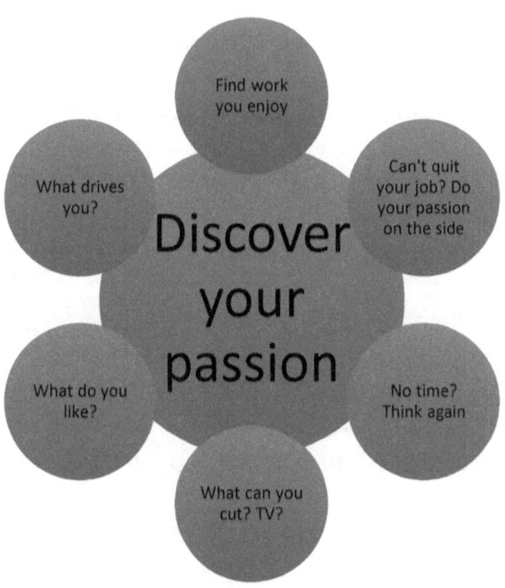

[13] *There is another serious problem I have seen under the sun. Hoarding riches harms the saver.* [14] *Money is put into risky investments that turn sour, and everything is lost. In the end, there is nothing left to pass on to one's children.* [15] *We all come to the end of our lives as naked and empty-handed as on the day we were born. We can't take our riches with us.*

[18] *Even so, I have noticed one thing, at least, that is good. It is good for people to eat, drink, and enjoy*

their work under the sun during the short life God has given them, and to accept their lot in life. [19] And it is a good thing to receive wealth from God and the good health to enjoy it. To enjoy your work and accept your lot in life—this is indeed a gift from God. [20] God keeps such people so busy enjoying life that they take no time to brood over the past." Ecclesiastes 5:10-16 NLT

King Solomon's Conclusion of the Matter

[24] So I decided there is nothing better than to enjoy food and drink and to find satisfaction in work. Then I realized that these pleasures are from the hand of God. [25] For who can eat or enjoy anything apart from him?

EXERCISING THE BODY

Obesity is of great concern in the United States and other countries. The Centers for Disease Control and Prevention (CDC) report that more than one-third of U.S. adults (35.7) are obese. The increase in obesity has led to several obesity-related conditions, including heart disease, strokes, type 2 diabetes, and certain types of cancers. In 2008, medical costs associated with obesity were estimated at $147 billion; the medical costs for people who are obese were $1,429 higher than those of normal weight.

Data from the National Health and Nutrition Examination Survey in April 2012, show that approximately 17% (12.5 million) of children and adolescents aged 2-19 years are obese. The prevalence of obesity among children and adolescents has almost tripled since 1980. We have a serious problem.

The UCLA Center for Human Nutrition presented a report that explains the benefits of physical activity and encourages us to become active. The Bible has been instructing us in that regard, for years:

"And every man that 'strives for the mastery' is temperate in all things..." [everyone who competes in the games goes into strict training..."] 1 Corinthians 9:25a

In Biblical times, there were competitive, Olympic-type games. The apostle Paul would not have said that *"they which run in a race run all but one receives the prize,"* (*1 Corinthians 9:24*) if he were not familiar with training and sport. The words "strive for the mastery," agonizomos," means "training for the Olympic games." ("Insight from the New Testament Greek," Biblefood.com)

"For physical training is of some value..." 1 Timothy 4:8

If you are not a gym person, there are many other recreational activities from which to choose. The following list is by no means exhaustive:

- Acting
- Air sports
- Archery
- Badminton
- Baking
- Baseball
- Basketball
- Beekeeping
- Biking
- Bird watching
- Boating
- Bowling
- Camping
- Candle making
- Canoeing
- Cooking
- Cricket
- Cycling
- Dancing
- Darts
- Fencing
- Field hockey
- Figure skating
- Fishing
- Flag football
- Flying
- Gardening
- Golfing
- Handball
- Hiking
- Horseback riding
- Ice hockey
- Jogging
- Juggling
- Jukskei
- Kayaking
- Kite flying
- Kitesurfing
- Lacrosse
- Longboarding
- Marbles
- Martial arts
- Metalworking
- Model building
- Motor sports
- Mountaineering
- Netball
- Paintball
- Playing musical instruments
- Polo
- Pottery
- Racquetball
- Rafting
- Rappelling
- Rock climbing
- Rugby
- Running
- Sailing
- Scuba diving
- Skating
- Skiing
- Skydiving
- Slot car racing
- Snow sports
- Squash
- Swimming
- Table football
- Table tennis
- Taekwondo
- Tai chi
- Tennis
- Topiary
- Triathlon
- Volleyball
- Walking
- Water sports
- Weightlifting
- Yoga
- Ziplining

CHAPTER 9

PRINCIPLES OF THE SOUL

'The soul is the seat of the emotions,' it is said. Defined as the spiritual part of a person, the mind is believed to give life to the body. It is credited with the faculties of thought and reasoning, action, and emotion. Almost everything that affects the body takes its cue from the soul.

Our modern world with all its conveniences and 'quick-fixes' is beset by stress. While stress has no face, its ravages are certainly seen in the human body. According to S.I. McMillen, author of None of These Diseases, "invisible emotional tension in the mind can produce striking visible changes in the body, changes that can become serious and fatal." [p. 58]

Stress has become the number one cause of doctor

visits. In 1948, statistics in the Journal of the American Medical Association revealed that two-thirds of patients who visited a doctor had symptoms and/or diseases that were caused or exacerbated by mental stress. (May 29, 1948, p. 442). Dr. S.I. McMillen stated that fear can deliver impulses along nerves from the emotional center to tighten the muscular outlet of the stomach. One of the results is that food might be prevented from passing into the intestines, resulting in regurgitation and stomach cramping and even diarrhea. (p. 57)

While the body can adapt to and deal with short-term stress, it was not designed to remain in this "flight or fight" mode for extended periods of time. If forced to do so, it begins to become vulnerable and may succumb to serious health issues. Death sometimes lurks not far behind. Some headaches occur as a result of anxiety. Discernible and indiscernible emotional tension in the body can lead to impaired memory and learning, elevated blood sugar levels and risk for diabetes, increased heartrate and other cardiovascular issues, respiratory immune, digestive, reproductive, and musculoskeletal problems. Worrying about an illness, consistently, can bring about the "self-fulfilling prophecy." The Bible teaches specifically about worry and stress and their effect on the body.

"A heart at peace gives life to the body," stated King Solomon (Prov. 14:30). It is so important for us to mentally entertain health, rather than illness, joy, rather than sorrow, and positivity, rather than its negative counterpart. The body mirrors the things on which the mind dwells. It is difficult to live wholly and happily, if our bodies are sluggish, sickly and unmotivated. The same thing is true of the soul and mind.

"Anxiety in a man's heart weighs him down, but a good word makes him glad." Proverbs 12:25

"The light of the eyes rejoices the heart: and a good report makes the bones fat" (healthy). Proverbs 15:30

Our conglomeration of beliefs and entertainment of them cause stress, which, leads to a breakdown of the body. Stress has been shown to cause strokes, high blood pressure, pain and clots in the heart; emotional tension can cause amenorrhea, dysmenorrhea, kidney disease, and even low libido.

It would behoove us well to alleviate our stress, or as much of it as we can. Being thankful, figuring out the cause of the concern and taking steps to resolve them will do much towards healing the soul.

EMOTIONAL HEALTH

The first step toward health is forgiveness.

I grew up hearing the phrase, "If you dig one pit, then you'd better dig two – one for your brother, yes and one for you." This bears out in the body and the mind. The vengeful, unforgiving desires within you will cut you down at the same time as it does your brother or sister, if not before.

The Word of God advises us against harboring

envy or holding grudges. Envy, jealousy, malice, pride (remember that little chorus?), unforgiveness, anger – all these emotions, when entertained and nurtured, eat away at the heart, both emotionally and physically, and become diseases. The book of Proverbs speaks to the dangers of these insidious, destructive emotions.

"A sound heart is the life of the flesh: but envy [is] the rottenness of the bones." Proverbs 14:30

We are also encouraged to make right those whom we have offended or whom we know may be offended because of us:

"Therefore, if you bring your gift to the altar, and there remember that your brother has ought (something) against you; leave there your gift before the altar, and go your way; first, be reconciled to your brother, and then come and offer your gift." Matthew 5:23-24

Having a cheerful disposition is important to the

healthy growth of the body, mind and spirit.

"A merry heart doeth good like a medicine: but a broken spirit dries the bones." Proverbs 17:22

"Heaviness in the heart of man makes it stoop: but a good word makes it glad." Proverbs 12:25

The verse, *"It is better to give than to receive,"* is bandied about rather conveniently. Many a time, these words are used when the speaker wants the listener to do something for him or give him something. This quote is actually a verse of Scripture, words given by the Lord Jesus.

In essence, we help ourselves when we help others. Helping others lifts our emotions, which in turn helps our entire being, body, mind, and soul.

A study was compiled by Peggy Thoits, along with Lyndi Hewitt from the Journal of Health and Social Behavior, in 2001, on the health benefits of helping others. Using a double wave panel study from the

Americans Changing Lives Study, Thoits and Hewitt studied 3,617 people, divided into two groups: those who volunteered and those who did not.

They studied the effects of volunteering on six different aspects of well-being, namely levels of happiness, life satisfaction, self-esteem; a sense of control over life, physical health, and depression. Thoits found that "volunteer work was good for both mental and physical health. People of all ages who volunteered were happier and experienced better physical health and less depression." The Corporation for National and Community Service reported that people who volunteer have lower depression rates, higher longevity, better functional ability, and lesser prevalence of heart disease.

Volunteering Lulls Chronic Pain

Paul Arnstein and some colleagues of Boston College conducted a study on the ways in which volunteering affected people who had chronic pain. The patients were evaluated on four levels: pain, disability, self-efficacy (the degree of confidence in the ability to control pain), and depression.

The findings revealed that "pain, depression, and disability decreased after volunteering, while self-efficacy remained stable." Over several months, Arnstein and his colleagues found that the "improvements continued without harm, suggesting that volunteering may help alleviate chronic pain."

Depression Derailed

Another study was performed by two researchers, Marc Musick and John Wilson, of the University of Texas at Austin. They used three years' worth of data from the Americans Changing Lives survey to learn the effects that volunteering had on depression. The respondents who had volunteered of their own volition, showed a lowering of depression, over time, for age groups. The act of volunteering, while being attributed with the lowered depression levels, was further heightened by the "social integration of volunteering."

*"Is not this the kind of fasting I have chosen:
7 Is it not to share your food with the hungry
and to provide the poor wanderer with shelter—
when you see the naked, to clothe them,
and not to turn away from your own flesh and blood?
8 Then your light will break forth like the dawn, and
your healing will quickly appear;
then your righteousness will go before you,
and the glory of the LORD will be your rear guard.
Isaiah 58:6-8 (NIV)*

SPIRITUAL CONNECTION

*Beloved, I wish above all things that thou mayest
prosper and be in health, even as thy soul prospers.
3 John 1:2 (KJV)*

There are several principles for health as applied to the spiritual man. Forgiveness is vital to healing. Scriptural nourishment is also essential (how else will we learn how to live our best life?)

Negativity breaks the body down. Practicing

uplifting thinking in spoken word and behavior are life and health-affirming. The best way to reverse negative thinking is to use the Scriptures, God's words.

> *Whatever things are true; whatever things are honest; whatever things are pure; whatever things are lovely; Whatever is admirable; if anything is excellent or praiseworthy, think about such things.*
> *Philippians 4:8*

In truth, we are emotional creatures, whether we think so or not. We pride ourselves on being tough and unmoved, but we were designed by God and His prototype links us with some commonalities. We feel love, hate, anger, joy, frustration, and sorrow, and we feel all the time. We sometimes allow the wrong emotions to saturate our minds. What we need to do is to be still and allow God to reorder the structure of our lives. His word remains constant; we should refer to it. His word is practical, we should read it. His word is fail-proof; we should implement it. In so doing, we will be at peace, even if the circumstances around us are in turmoil.

We will be rested, hydrated, stress-less individuals who have learnt to listen to our own body language.

"If you pay attention to these laws and are careful to follow them, then the Lord your God will… keep you free from every disease." Deuteronomy 7:12, 15

CHAPTER 12

REFUSE THE REFUSE

"You must have a designated area outside the camp where you can go to relieve yourself. Each of you must have a spade as part of your equipment. Whenever you relieve yourself, dig a hole with the spade and cover the excrement."

"You shall have a place outside the camp, and you shall go out to it. And you shall have a trowel with your tools, and when you sit down outside, you shall dig a hole with it and turn back and cover up your excrement."   *Deuteronomy 23:12-13*

What happens to our bodily refuse after we flush in a rush? If we were to be obedient, then our refuse would be buried, thereby lessening our incidence of disease and increase in our death numbers. Unfortunately, this is not the case.

The Portland Mercury details quite clearly the process that our refuse undergoes after it leaves our bodies and goes down the toilet. It joins with rain water, garbage, chemical pollutants like household cleaners, biological contaminants and other refuse in the sewers and then goes through a series of sifting and chlorination until what is determined to be "clean water" is reached.

The thicker, sifted material is transported to the dump; the "clean water' is poured into our cisterns and appear with a gush into our sinks, tubs, pots, and upon our bodies when we open our taps. Our feces and urine are recycled into our very bodies. We are drinking the very source of our disease and degeneration. The chlorine, yet another chemical, and a dangerous one at that, merely adds to our degeneration. Fluoride is then added, supposedly to strengthen bones and teeth, but really, more as a taste enhancer.

[Source: What happens to our bodily refuse after we send it down the toilet? The Sordid Life of Human Waste. http://www.portlandmercury.com/portland/where-does-my-poop-go/Content?oid=28160.]

Inattention to health and waste disposal has proven detrimental. Innovation has brought an increase in the amount of household waste that is generated daily. Our waste is combined into municipal waste collection and then transported to landfill sites. Of course, we know that if waste is not properly disposed of, it will become a health hazard.

"Different methods of waste management emit a large number of substances. Raised incidence of low birth weight births has been related to residence near landfill sites, as has the occurrence of various congenital malformations... Studies of cancer incidence and mortality in populations around landfill sites or incinerators have been equivocal, with varying results for different cancer sites."

Oxford Academic British Medical Bulletin, https://academic.oup.com/bmb/article/68/1/183/421368

CHAPTER 13

BIBLICAL HEALTH, UNDENIABLY CONTROVERSIAL; UNDENIABLY UNDENIABLE

The Bible is and has always been a book that sparks controversy. The controversy occurs because people either have not read it in its entirety, thereby misunderstanding its truths, or they are offended because it upholds a level of morality to which they have no desire to adhere. As such, some try to cast aspersions on the Scriptures because it causes a soul pricking which they cannot ignore.

What they do not realize is that God's laws are intended to bless His people. Though given initially to the Children of Israel, the instructions are quite beneficial and life-changing to all of us. As Dr. Rex Russell put it, "this blessing was not just a spiritual blessing; it was a holistic blessing, including the Jewish people's health and social structure. (What the Bible Says About Healthy Living. P.8)

The Hebrew word *shalom* means peace, welfare, blessing in all aspects of life." What is the best way to know true health? Live by the Bible. It is that simple. The Bible's teachings are not just for believers. Anyone, by following the principles of the Bible, will benefit from God's instructions for healthy living.

> *"If you listen carefully to the voice of the Lord your God and do what is right in his eyes, if you pay attention to his commands and keep all his decrees, I will not bring on you any of the diseases I brought on the Egyptians, for I am the Lord, who heals you."*
> *Exodus 15:26*

What were some of the diseases that the Egyptians suffered? According to Dr. Rex Russell, radiographs and autopsies by paleo pathologists, on Egyptian mummies showed evidence of vascular disease, arthritis, tooth decay, infections, cancer, emphysema, tuberculosis, parasites, pneumonia, and obesity. Mummified Pharaohs, Russell noted, often show the most advanced degenerative diseases. Historically, Pharaohs and other royalty were the only ones whose diets included large quantities of meat and delicacies."

> *[King] Solomon's daily provisions were thirty cors of the finest flour and sixty cors of meal, ten head of stall-fed cattle and a hundred sheep and goats, as well as deer, gazelles, roebucks and choice fowl." 1 Kings 4:22*

There are some creatures that God created for human consumption and are non-toxic. The others are toxic and were not created for our consumption.

Dr. Rex Russell reported the results of a study by Dr. David Macht of Johns Hopkins University, in 1953. Dr. Macht studied the "toxic effects of animal flesh on a controlled growth culture. A substance was classified as toxic if it slowed the culture's growth rate below 75%. According to Dr. Russell, the results of Dr. Macht's study showed that "the lower the growth percentage of the culture, the more toxic the flesh."

Dr. Macht's results were posted in the following table. The table clearly shows that we are eating many toxic substances that were not created for food. Of the creatures listed in the table, the ones that have a percentage above 75 are nontoxic or clean. The animals that do not have percentage rankings were not studied but Dr. Macht included them in order to provide a more comprehensive list of clean and unclean meats:

Clean and Unclean Meats

(Any number below 75% is toxic — See text for explanation)

Four-Footed Animals

CLEAN		UNCLEAN	
(Cloven-hoofed, cud-chewing)		(All others)	
calf	82%	black bear	59%
deer	98%	camel	41%
goat	90%	cat	62%
ox	91%	coney (guinea pig)	46%
sheep	94%	dog	62%
		fox (silver)	58%
		grizzley bear	55%
		ground hog	53%
		hamster	46%
		horse	39%
		opossum	53%
		rabbit	49%
		rat	55%
		rhinoceros	60%
		squirrel	43%
		swine (pigs/hogs)	54%

TheHerbDoc™

Flying Animals

CLEAN		UNCLEAN	
goose	85%	bat	
chicken	83%	cormorant	
coot	88%	crow	46%
duck	98%	eagle	
pigeon	93%	falcon	
quail	89%	hawk	
swan	87%	heron	
turkey	85%	ibis	
		kite	
		nighthawk	
		osprey	
		ostrich	
		owl	62%
		pelican	
		raven	
		red-tail hawk	36%
		sparrow hawk	36%
		sea gull	
		stork	
		vulture	

Water Creatures

CLEAN		UNCLEAN	
(With scales and fins)		(Without scales and fins)	
black bass	80%	catfish	48%
black drum	105%	clams	
bluefish	80%	crabs	
carp	90%	eel	40%
channel bass	80%	lobster	
chub	91%	octopus	
cod	98%	oysters	
croaker	90%	porcupine fish	60%
flounder	83%	puffer	51%
flying fish	87%	sand skate	59%
goldfish	88%	scallops	
haddock	80%	shark (dogfish)	62%
hake	98%	shrimp	
halibut	82%	squid	
herring	100%	stingray	46%
kingfish	83%	toad fish	49%
mullet	87%		
pike	98%		
pompano	110%		
porgy	80%		
rainbow trout	81%		
rock bass	100%		
salmon	81%		
smelt	90%		
sea bass	103%		
shad	100%		
Spanish mackerel	98%		
spot	80%		
sturgeon	87%		
tuna (bluefin)	88%		
white perch	81%		
whiting, Carolina	84%		
yellow perch	87%		

Insects

CLEAN	UNCLEAN
(Winged, with jointed hopping legs)	(All others)
cricket	
grasshopper	
katydid	
locust	

Source: Abundant Life Herb Shop

The Whole Truth

Dr. Bernard Jensen stated that the "health of body and mind and spirit derives from proper food, correct living and high thoughts… a very simple concept but one frequently overlooked."

For many, our bodies are being broken down through years of abuse, which has led to ailments and disease. Diseases, from the seemingly innocuous cold, to the feared cancer, ravage our bodies. Our environment, polluted air, genetically modified foods, irradiated foods also add to the breakdown of our bodies, further making them vulnerable to disease.

If we begin to take the time to feed ourselves with

the right foods, as outlined in the Bible, rest well, hydrate, exercise and pursue peace, we will do much towards improving and maintaining good health. The body will then continue its process of self-healing. That is, after all, the way that the Great Architect designed it.

Who knows us better than the One who created us? Contained within the pages of the Bible are all the things that pertain to life. Let us seek life and live.

Dear Friend,

Do you know that God wants you to be well and at peace? He loves you so very much. His Word, the Bible, reveals His love and yearning over you.

"The LORD has appeared of old to me, saying: 'Yes, I have loved you with an everlasting love; Therefore with loving-kindness I have drawn you.'" Jeremiah 31:3 (NKJV)

He wants you to be well in your mind, body, and spirit. He wants you to care for your body with proper exercise, diet, and rest; He wants you to take care of your mind by alleviating stress, and addressing emotionally oppressive issues.

"Guard your heart above all else, for it determines the course of your life." Proverbs 4:23 (NLT)

God also wants you to take care of your spirit. He invites you to share a personal relationship with Him through His Son, the Lord Jesus. If you have not met Him, know that this can only be done by accepting Jesus Christ as your Lord and Savior.

Say this prayer to Him, with sincerity:

Dear God,

I believe that you love me and sent your Son, Jesus Christ, to die for my sins. I receive You, now, as my Lord and Savior. Thank You for saving me. Please take control of my life. I look to You to help me to live the way You want me to live. Amen.

Congratulations and welcome to the family!

If you don't own a Bible, try to obtain one. It is God's love letter to you. Talk to Jesus, your new friend, often, and ask Him to lead you to a church where you can learn more about Him.

Lesa Lawson, ND, HHC
Naturopathic Doctor

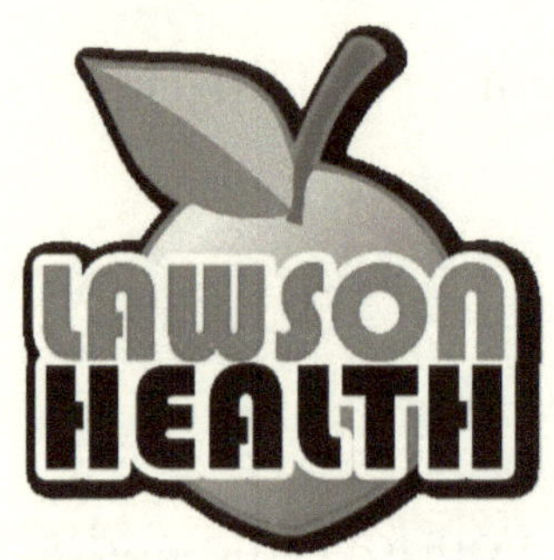

LawsOnHealth Wellness

102 Dry Mill Road; Unit 102
Leesburg, VA 20175
(571) 252-3428
lawsonhealth@gmail.com
lawsonhealthwellness.com

Your Health Matters

Also by Dr. Lesa Lawson…

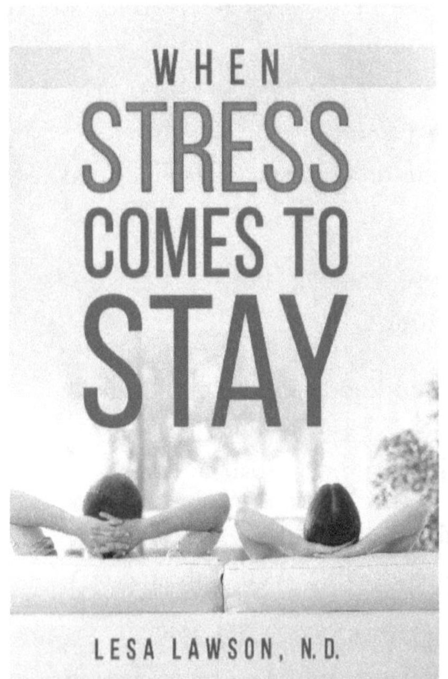

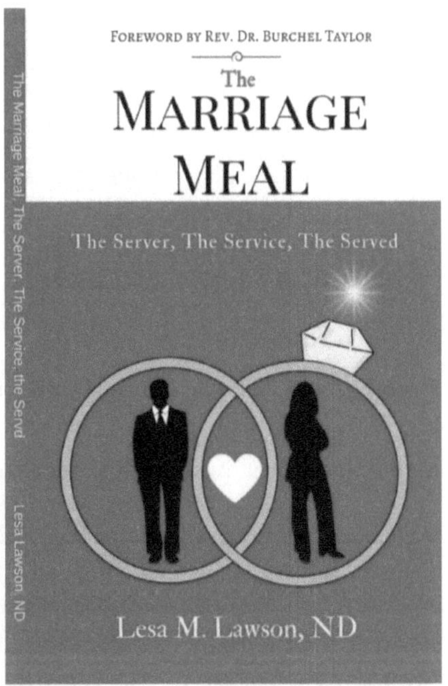

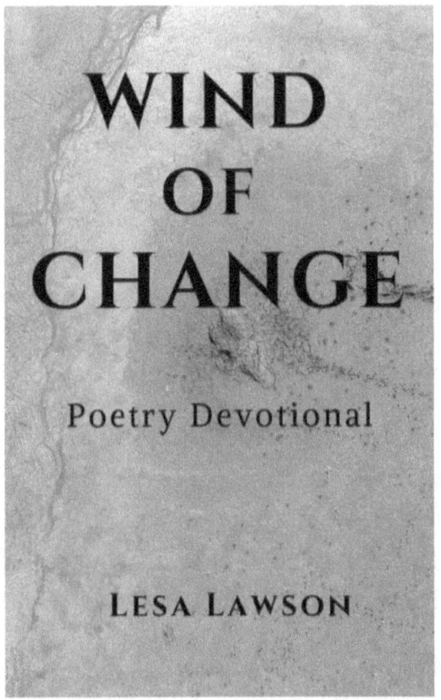

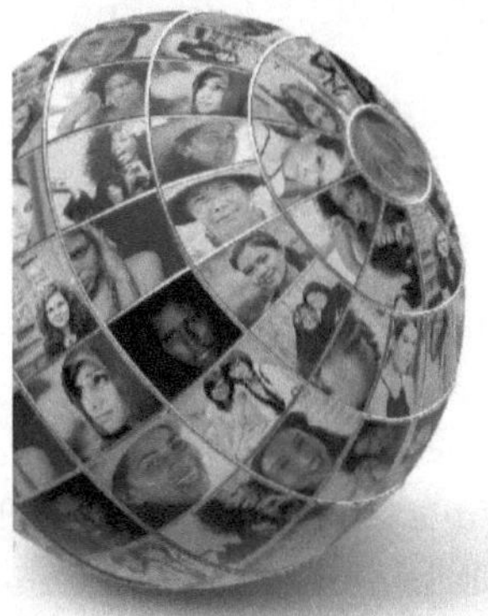

Works Cited

Acid Alkaline Food Chart with 12 Perfect Foods
http://www.acidalkalinediet.com/alkaline-foods-list/acid-alkaline-food-chart-with-12-perfect-foods

Anthony, Richard, Biblical Health Principles.
http://www.ecclesia.org/truth/health.html

Coal Tar For Breakfast? The Truth Behind Food Additives,
http://recipes.howstuffworks.com/coal-tar-breakfast-additives.htm
http://www.healthychild.org/issues/chemical-pop/Coal_tar_dyes/

Fairchild, Mary, Foods of the Bible: Bible Foods with Scripture References.
New York: The New York Times Company, 2012. Web. <about.com>.

Food and Agriculture Organization of the United Nations:
http://www.fao.org/docrep/t0690e/t0690e06.htm. Accessed September 3,
2012

Guzik, David, Leviticus 11 - Clean and Unclean Animals, *2004.*
http://www.enduringword.com/commentaries/0311.htm

Henry, Matthew, Matthew Henry's Commentary, Zondervan/ Marshall,
Morgan & Scott, Ltd. 1961. Print.

Kashrut: Jewish Dietary Laws. http://www.jewfaq.org/kashrut.htm.
Accessed September 1, 2012
http://www.jewishvirtuallibrary.org/jsource/Judaism/species.html

Kilmer, Chris, Hand Washing Rate Low Among Doctors, Oct. 21, 2009.
http://abcnews.go.com/2020/superfreakonomics-dirty-hands-deadly-infections/story?id=8861823&singlePage=true#.UCgOp6FlRDc]. Last
reviewed June 2012 by Brian Randall, MD. 2008 EBSCO Publishing. 2012
Beth Israel Deaconess Medical Center. Boston, MA 02215

Lowe, Henry, *Exotic Teas, The Caribbean and the Rest of the World.* Kingston 5,

Jamaica, W.I., Pelican Publishers Limited, 2007. Print

McMillen, M.D., S.I. *None of These Diseases*. Grand Rapids, MI: Fleming H. Revell/ Baker Book House Company, 1963. Print.

National Center for Biotechnology Information, U.S. National Library of Medicine 8600 Rockville Pike, Bethesda MD, 20894 USA. http://www.ncbi.nlm.nih.gov/pubmed/18261540

Post, G.E. *Bible Dictionary Contributions*. Thayer's Lexicon: ζιζάνια. Old Dominion University. http://www.odu.edu/~lmusselm/plant/bible/allbibleplantslist.php

Shelton, Herbert M, M.D. *The Hygienic System: Orthotrophy*, Dr. Shelton's Health School. 1975, 1935. http://chestofbooks.com/health/natural-cure/The-Hygienic-System-Orthotrophy/index.html#ixzz29DrLw35V

Shimer, Katie, What happens to our bodily refuse after we send it down the toilet? The Sordid Life of Human Waste. http://www.portlandmercury.com/portland/where-does-my-poop-go/Content?oid=28160.

Stowe, Faye C. *The Whole Woman*. Kansas City: Beacon Hill Press, 1984. Print.

Strong, LL.D., S.T.D., James. *The New Strong's Exhaustive Concordance of the Bible*. Nashville, Tennessee: Thomas Nelson Publishers, 1996. Print.

Strueh, Kurt. "Parasites in Swine." Purdue University, n.d. Web. 4 Oct 2012. <www.extension.purdue.edu/pork/health/kurtstrueh.html>.

The Holy Bible, Authorized King James Version. Thomas Nelson, Inc., 2003. Print. www.ThomasNelson.com.

Thoits PA, Hewitt LN. Volunteer work and well-being. *Journal of Health and Social Behavior*. 2001;42:115-131.

Thoits, Peggy A. , Hewitt, Lyndi N. , Vanderbilt University Journal of Health and Social Behavior, 2001, Vol. 42 (June): 115-131.

UCLA Center for Human Nutrition.
http://www.cellinteractive.com/ucla/nutrition_101/phys_lect5b.html.
Accessed. August 31, 2012

Uses of Gelatin.
http://www.gelatininnovations.com/pages/uses_of_gelatin.html. Last
updated: April 30, 2009. Accessed: September 1, 2012

Volunteering in the United States, 2011. United States Department of
Labor, Bureau of Labor Statistics. Available
at: http://www.bls.gov/news.release/volun.toc.htm . Published February
22, 2012. Accessed June 18, 2012.

Zohary, M. (1982) *Plants of the Bible*. New York: Cambridge University Press,
Liddell H G and Scott R, *A Greek-English Lexicon*, Clarendon Press, Oxford,
1843–1996, under "ζιζάνια".

Images: Pixabay.com

ABOUT THE AUTHOR

Lesa Lawson, ND is a Naturopathic Doctor and Colon Hydrotherapist. Her practice is firstly, integrative (blending age-old healing traditions with scientific advances and current research). Secondly, it is holistic (treating with a number of mental and social factors which impact human health negatively).

Dr. Lawson specializes in alternative therapies that help clients regain their digestive health. Her area of focus is the gut / stomach as it is the seat of most illnesses arising from factors such as poor diet, dehydration, medications interacting negatively with one another, stress, or unhealthy working or living environments.

Her personal and professional health journey led to a profound appreciation for healing from the inside out. She continues to do research in Jamaica and the United States. Not satisfied simply with apprising herself of information and because her practice is one in which she, along with her clients, are partners in their health, she educates readily, conducting seminars in Jamaica and the United States.

She is the founder of LawsOnHealth Wellness, a haven of healing located in Northern Virginia. Dr. Lawson's first work is the thought-provoking, *Six Lies Women Believe about Their Health*, followed by *When Stress Comes to Stay*, *Wind of Change*, and *The Marriage Meal*.